# SUNRISE

## DAOIST PRACTICES FOR WOMEN

Caryn Boyd Diel

Village Books Publishing
BELLINGHAM, WASHINGTON

DRAGON
FIRE
PRODUCTIONS

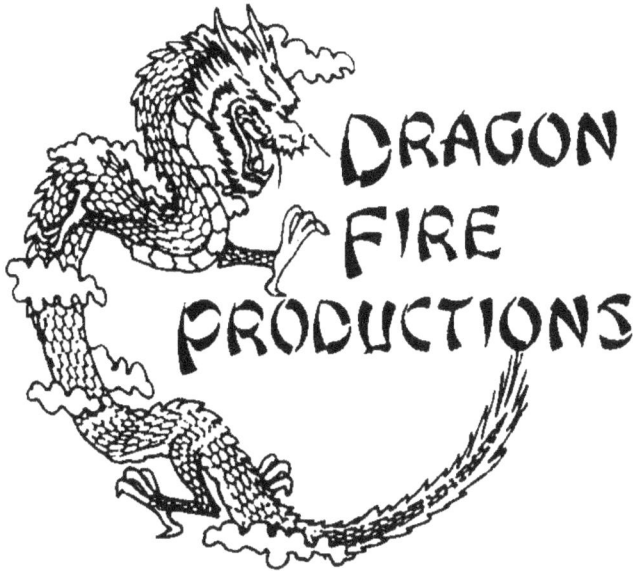

Village Books Publishing
1200 11th St, Bellingham, WA 98225
Bellingham, WA 98225
publishing@villagebooks.com

Disclaimer: No part of this book should be used to replace the medical advice of your doctor.

Book Layout ©2017 BookDesignTemplates.com

Sunrise: Daoist Practices for Women/ Caryn Boyd Diel. -- 1st ed.
ISBN 978-1-7338695-2-2

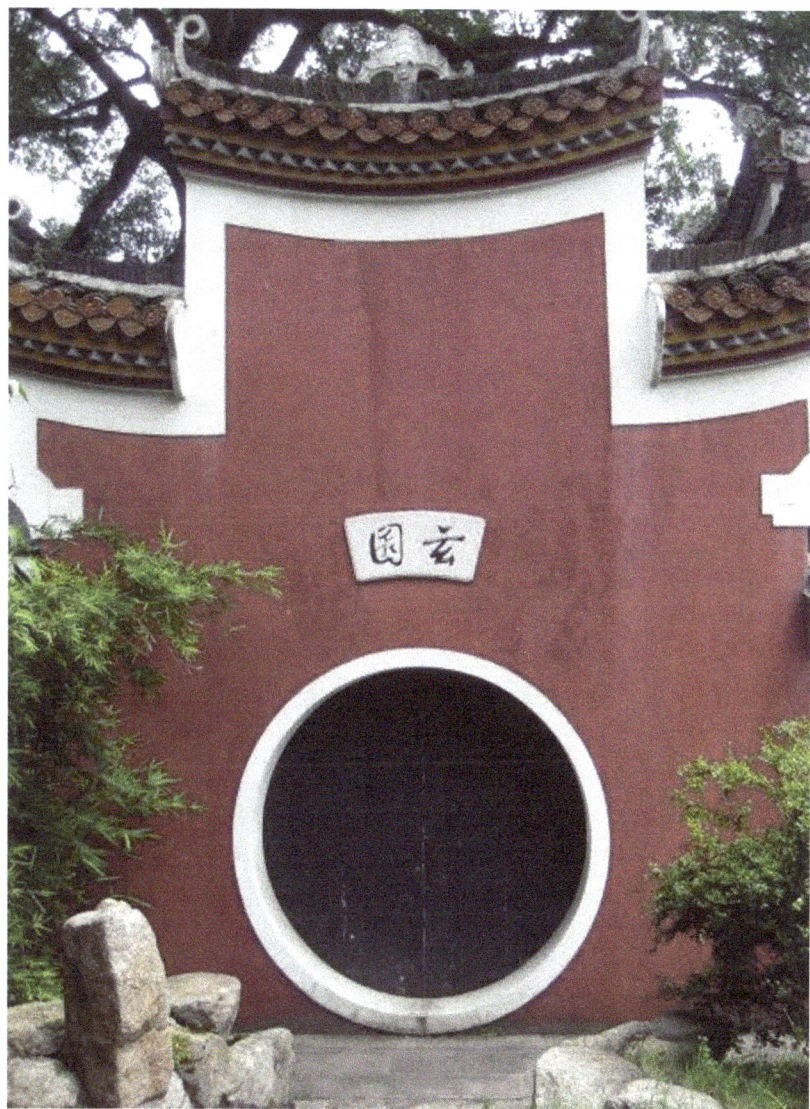

## *FOREWORD*

I have divided this manual of Daoist practices for Women into 3 sections: Curing and Healing, Yang Shen: Prevention and Longevity, and Immortality practices.

You will find several Daoist practices in Section 1 which will positively affect behaviors and lifestyle choices, leading you into the experience of balance and healing. Section 2 expands and supports your healing practices, guiding you to a healthy long life, yang shen; longevity. It is a rare individual who will choose to incorporate the immortality practices into their life, however, that is also your option. In Section 3 I outline some of the classic Daoist immortality practices and ways of seeking guidance; these are ancient and profound. It takes dedication and a complete lack of expectation as to how long this might take to achieve. It is a path one chooses. The Dao is a path of personal dedication to inner growth and awareness, which is aligned with all nature. The pace of nature is patience, the lesson is simplicity and stillness; trusting the Dao of Heaven and Earth.

Practice for 100 days nurtures your kidney chi

300 days is the foundation for immortal medicine

2 years your body will become light and your mind effective

3 years is the foundation for ascending to reach the undefinable truth

"Look at a tree, a flower, a plant. Let your awareness rest upon it. How still they are, how deeply rooted in Being. Allow nature to teach you stillness"

–ECKHART TOLLE, A MODERN DAY MYSTIC

# Contents

# Introduction

The Dao is a path one chooses, a path of nature, which is sometimes fluid like water, and other times requires stamina like hiking a mountain.

*"Actualization of our Life's Destiny is achieved through internal Alchemy, which is one of the paths of the Tao"*

-Sun Bu'er (1119-1182)

**Female Shaman**
Daoist Practices have historically been held as precious information and kept alive in the deepest parts of mountain caves and grottos. Men and Women have shared quietly of what they knew, passing along instructions orally from master to student for centuries. Shamanic cultures prize natural places for the purity of chi that is found there, and are guided by the changing of the seasons. Daoism represents an ancient way of relating to all of nature and the heavens above as the guiding truth of the Dao. The human body revealed itself to ancient practitioners as a microcosm of the macrocosmic universe.

Daoist practices are deeply imbedded in the manifestation of spiritual knowledge into the material plane; the redemption of spirit through meditation and longevity practices. The human body, in every cell, is the recipient and transforming vehicle of the practices. Daoist alchemy cannot live on a piece of paper or in a book. Daoism is not fully alive unless it is flowing through all nature, including women and men.

**What is Daoism?**
Daoism has its roots in a Shamanic society 5-10,000 years ago. The Wu shaman of the past were primarily women. There are clay images of them dancing and bringing rain, healing, calling in the spirits. Lao Tze called the Dao, the Great Mother of all things. The Dao translates as the void, which is nothingness but encompasses everything. To follow a Daoist path is to follow the natural laws of the universe. Matter, Chi/energy and Space create a universe. They balance each other like yin and yang; one defines the other.

Daoism is the indigenous philosophy of China and embraces the cosmology of the Natural world, which sees our body as a microcosm of the whole. As we adapt Daoist practices into our modern day lives we reach back at the same time that we look forward. Daoism is about adapting to change. Change has come quickly in our lives and therefore Daoism can provide guidance and peace of mind about the true nature of things.

Daoism is compatible with all occupations. One does not need to be a hermit, a nun or a recluse. As the Dao exists in all things, human and nature, living in accordance with the virtue of non-interference and cultivation of inner peace is easily supported in any society, and any culture. Supporting health and surrendering to life is simply returning to source, like each drop of heavenly rain returns to the ocean.

"In the West, the stage for Taoism's entry was first set by the lifestyles and beliefs of the Native Americans (the West's original Taoists). Not unlike Mao and his band of thugs, who sought to annihilate Taoism in China, the co-called Christian White Man tried viciously to eradicate the American Indian way of life. ...Henry David Thoreau made a great contribution by writing Walden.... In the way that Taoism always does, it glides through this open gate, entering slowly, quietly, and almost without notice. ...the free thinking associated with Taoist thought is appealing to many westerners." Stuart Alve Olson. *The Jade Emperors Minds Seal Classic.*

Our fast moving culture needs the simplicity that Daoism offers.

Virtue is a manifestation of the Dao, which guides beliefs and behaviors. The goal of the Dao is stillness and the application of that is simplicity. There are many practices in this book which may require you to learn things which change your beliefs and behaviors. At the beginning most female practitioners feel that they are overwhelmed by the amount of tasks they already tackle on a daily basis. "How and when do I fit these new self-care practices into my life?" "When do I find the time to meditate?" I can tell you that the inner peace, increased level of chi and radiant health that you experience from Daoist practices will create a passion inside of you to devote yourself to making practice a priority.

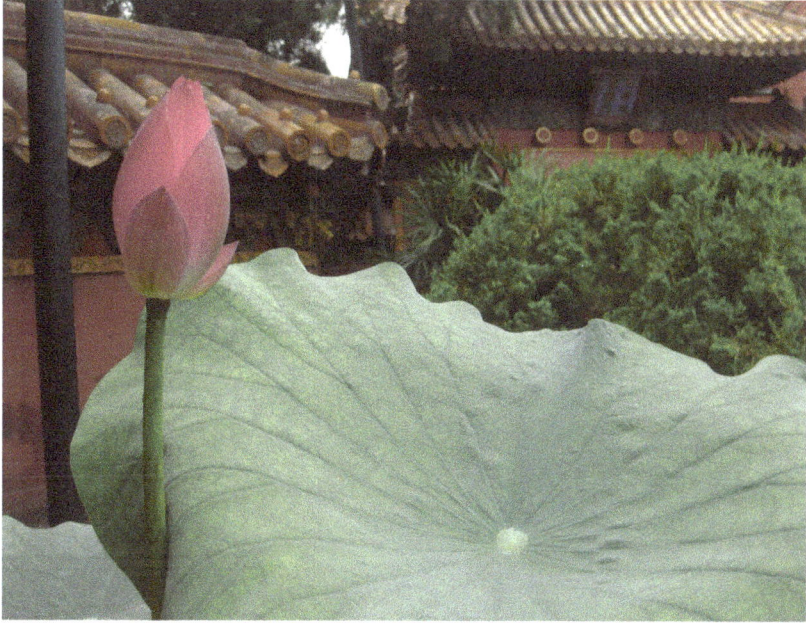

# SECTION 1

# Curing & Healing

Healing brings life into balance and harmony. When you experience healing, life unfolds as meaningful and productive you are able to cultivate virtue and inner peace. Healing brings you to a new sense of completion, not a return to what was before.

Curing eliminates symptoms which may lead to disease, or symptoms which have already manifested as disease. You may need to seek the help of others in either curing or healing.

Historically Chinese doctors only received payment if their patients stayed healthy, the emphasis being on prevention, harmony and balance. What we eat, how we work, exercise, relax, interact with family and society, sleep, how we handle our emotions and our sexual behaviors are all important in keeping balance and vitality.

Sun Sumiao was a famous traditional Chinese medicine doctor of the Sui and Tang dynasty. Named China's 'King of Medicine' for his significant contributions to Chinese medicine, Sun Sumiao displayed tremendous care for his patients and left us with instructions on Health, Diet, Meditation and Immortality. He coined the term Ashi points. Ashi points are used in acupuncture and massage. Sun Sumiao lived from 581 AD - 682 AD. He was called the master of subtle resonance.

*His advice: Ask yourself, "What is right with me?" What makes my life pleasurable? Do not focus on the disease process but on what make your life meaningful.*

There are too many choices today, numerous healing modalities and competing belief systems. In which one do you have the most confidence and faith? Who supports your expectations of getting well? The way of Daoist health is to simplify and find stillness in life. Face what destiny brings to you with your eyes open and move through it.

Nourish Life, embrace the bad and the good. Step away from the bad when you can. The Daoist point of view is that suffering is relative to who you are and how you experience life. Never allow wounds to be nurtured. Embrace them and learn from them, however, don't become the victim. Everything is relative and comparable in duality like, tai chi. Change is the rhythm of life. Look at patterns. The wisdom of the I Ching (book of changes) is to see patterns in our life and to develop a good attitude and the right timing to make progress smooth. The Dao provokes change. Be mindful of what your body wants you to honor. Listen to your body. The Daoist point of view is that the body is as important as the mind.

**The Key to Longevity is what you do now.**

In Section 1 there are practices that you could adopt if healing from an illness. Many of the "Curing and Healing" practices are also fine Longevity practices. If a specific practice brings healing or curing into your life, then you may decide to continue with it for the benefits it offers. There are some topics not included here as the scope of them is too large to cover adequately. Herbs, Acupuncture, Oils and Stone Medicine (healing with crystals and ground stones) are integral methods of healing in Traditional Chinese Medicine. There are many books and practitioners who excel in these healing modalities. Seek them out in your area if you are drawn to experience them.

# Inner Smile Meditation

How do you feel when someone smiles authentically to you? Contact that feeling inside of yourself and feel the responsive smile beginning in your face and spreading out to your ears and into your eyes. Now let that smile melt through your entire body filling every cell. Sense the cells expanding and relaxing, becoming clear and spacious.

The practice of Inner Smile meditation raises the frequency of the cells in your body. Joy is a non-dual frequency, it exists in a higher dimension than the emotions that arise from the organs in the body. As you raise the frequency of every cell you bring a healing vibration into your body. One of the reasons that we seek various experiences or foods or sex, or whatever it is that one craves, it is to shift the vibration in our body to something happy. This happy state does not last forever, or long enough to satisfy us, and so we continue to seek and to re-create the feeling.

The inner smile meditation is one way to re-create that feeling of happiness, a lifted frequency, in our bodies. It is expansive and very good for us. If your brain thinks that you are happy, then it creates happy chemistry which spreads through the body. If you can successfully bring a smile into just one cell, you have created a change for the better.

*The Inner Smile is a classic example of a Daoist meditation. Simple yet profound.*

The practice is simple; sit for a few minutes and begin to feel deeply into a memory of smiling whole-body happiness. It is important that you actually bring a smile to your face to re-create the feeling in your body. Or perhaps you want to create a new experience and can imagine that feeling, do this several times a day until you become good at shifting your vibration to a high frequency of joy.

The Inner Smile is a traditional beginning to the Six Healing Sounds meditation. We smile into the organs prior to bringing color and sound into the body. This practice is simple and also included in the section of this book as a longevity practice because it is so beneficial.

# The 6 Healing Sounds

The practice of the six healing sounds for nourishing a healthy life has a long oral and written history. During the Qin Dynasty (221-207 BC) there was a record of this practice and in the Han Dynasty (207 BC- 220 AD) we find written records buried in tombs. In the Tang dynasty (618-906AD) Sun Si Miao, and esteemed TCM doctor, wrote in the "Song of Hygiene" about the six healing sounds and outlined their specific benefits to the internal organs and their associated sense organs.

Healing practices that were passed down orally for centuries were eventually recorded on silk and bamboo and later unearthed in tombs. Many modern day practitioners in China know of this practice and when I was in China in 2011 I met a Taoist Abbot who told me that this was, indeed, an advanced practice. He stressed the need to make the sounds gently and sub-vocally. Clearly the most basic practices are advanced practices, affording the practitioner immediate internal alchemical results. This is a classic Taoist foundation practice in that the most simple of practices become the most profound.

This practice is flexible and adaptable to each individual's needs. You may practice them in order, (starting with Wood and proceeding through the creation cycle, ending with the endocrine or triple burner sound) or only practice the sounds you need to treat specific conditions in the body. I like to focus my practice seasonally, meaning that in spring I would give specific focus to the Wood element and the Liver sound.

Many esteemed Taoist sages advised that the first step in practice is to subdue one's emotions, and then to harmonize the mind. Chen Tuan marks these as the first 3 of 12 steps to attain the Tao.

**Sun Buer**

*Be free from grief and
    anxiety.
A solitary cloud and wild
    crane beyond constraint.
Within a thatched hut,
Leisurely read the golden
    books.
Forests and streams outside
    the window,
At the edge of the rolling
    hills, water and bamboo.
Luminous moon and clear
    wind;
Become worthy to be their
    companion.*

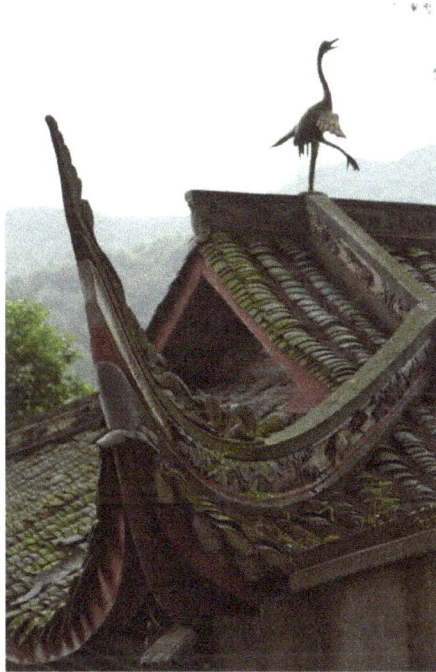

Daoist practitioners realize that humans have desires and emotions and they provided us with alchemical formulas to transform this energy into pure chi.

As a healing practice the Six Healing Sounds meditation is unequaled in its ability to identify dense emotional energy/chi in the body; specifically in each organ, and to then diffuse it and break up patterns of stagnation which form disease and behavior problems. Communicating with color and sound to clear and tonify the organ's chi is a very old archetype of healing. You are connecting to the subtle energy/chi field by using your ability to visualize and guide the chi with sound and color. This practice recycles chi into its original pure form therefore bringing balance and harmony back into the body mind as is was in a primordial state.

If you are restoring your health it is important for every cell to be functioning at a high level of clarity, unencumbered with emotional toxins. The environment of the cell, the cell wall, is affected by your thoughts, emotions, and sounds. Women, pay close attention to the Sounds and Color used in this practice for balancing and strengthening the endocrine glands.

Sound and Color are ancient archetypes of healing. Sound breaks up stagnation and patterns of disease, in this case stuck emotions. Color tonifies the cells of the body. True colors signify vibrant health. See the above 5 elements graph to see the colors. (the Metal element color is White)

We begin the 6 healing sounds meditation with the Inner Smile practice which lifts the frequency in the cells to a higher vibration. Then visualize each organ filling with a pure color that is associated with it's element. The sounds will purge any low vibration emotion from the body. (the sounds are always sub vocal, like a whisper) For the Fire element the sound is Haaaaa. Feel the sound emanating from the heart and small intestines, removing stagnation. The sound for the Earth element is Hooooo, very guttural. Metal element sound is Sssssssss. Water element sound is Choooooooo, like a wave crashing. Feel the contraction in your core around the kidneys as you make this sound. Wood element sound is Shhhhhhhh.

The 6th healing sound is for the Endocrine glands; pituitary, pineal, thyroid, thymus, adrenal, pancreas, ovaries and testes. The color with will tonify them is a deep night sky violet/purple. The sound is Heeeeeeeee. The virtuous behavior that comes from balanced endocrine glands is effortless and harmonious communication.

Practice in class with a teacher, or listen to the CD which is included in this manual. You may want to watch it the first time through (track 1 on the CD). Both tracks are real time meditations. Practice at least once a day, more if you are recovering from illness. Doing the 6 healing sounds before bedtime is excellent for harmonizing the organs' chi and assisting you to sleep peacefully. Do this meditation daily to clear your body/mind of low vibrations.

This is a foundation practice which will prepare you for other practices.

The graph below explains which organs manifest specific emotions. It also shows you which color is used to tonify the organs. (the color used to tonify the Metal element is White)The second graph will show you which seasons are associated with the organs.

The endocrine glands are included in the 6 healing sounds, and in the 24 hour meridian cycle they are active in the late evening, but have no season.

Daoist considered the hormones to be "spirit molecules"; very fine and very powerful, and were therefore given the color Purple to match the North Star.

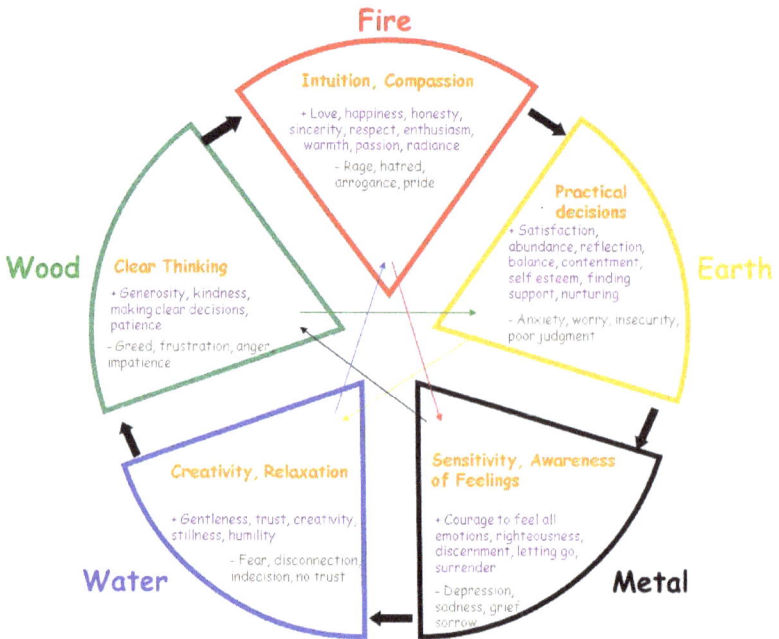

*C 2001 Caryn Diel*

The graph illustrates the Positive emotions in Purple, negative emotions in brown. Orange signifies the mental state of being and behaviors that come from having balanced emotions.

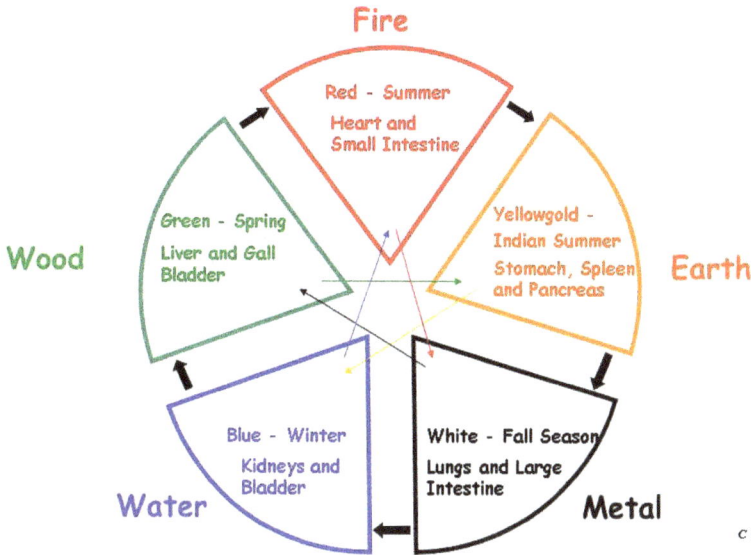

Fire

Red - Summer
Heart and
Small Intestine

Green - Spring
Liver and Gall
Bladder

Wood

Yellowgold –
Indian Summer
Stomach, Spleen
and Pancreas

Earth

Blue - Winter
Kidneys and
Bladder

White - Fall Season
Lungs and Large
Intestine

Water

Metal

C 2001 Caryn Diel

The 5 seasons and the 5 Elements as they relate to the paired organs. It is wise to be mindful of the organs during their associated season. Nurture them with the proper foods and qigong practices. Slow down in the Winter, rest more.

The 6 Healing Sounds practice is useful in healing and it is also a Long Life/Yang Shen practice. One of my teachers, Master Mantak Chia, claims that this practice will cool down the organs' chi and allow the body to be more at ease. Emotions affect the organs, and unhealthy organs create unhealthy emotions.

# TIMETABLE OF MERIDIANS

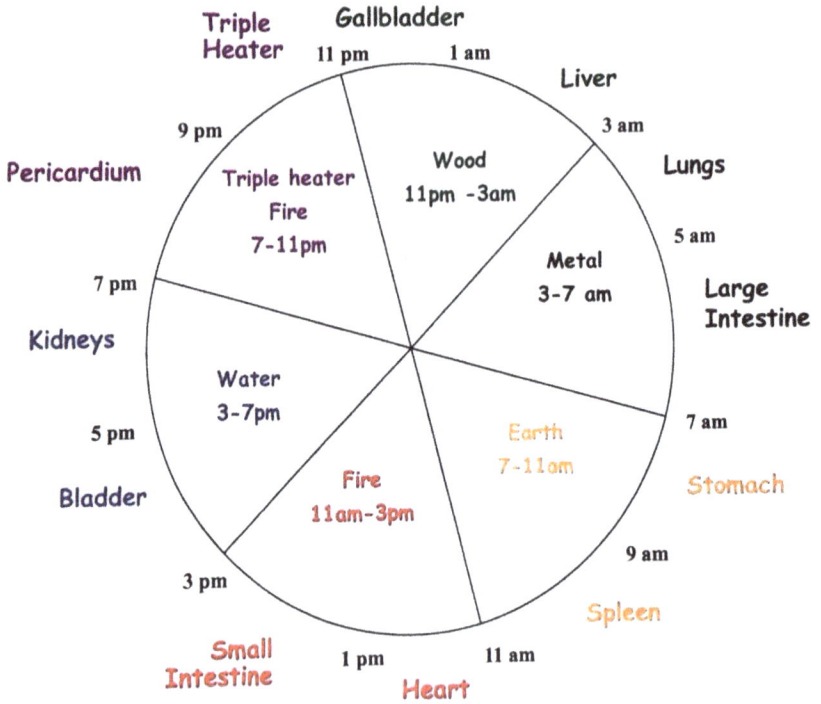

## THE ELEMENTS, THE HIGHER VIRTUES AND THE SOUNDS

**Metal Element**
Lungs and Large Intestine, SSSSSSSSSSS
Fall
White
Virtues: Courage, Sensitivity to feelings, Righteousness, Discernment, letting go, surrender
Negative aspects: Sadness, Grief, Depression

**Water Element**
Kidneys and Bladder, CHOOOOOO (like the sound of waves crashing)
Winter
Dark Blue
Virtues: Gentleness, Trust, Stillness, Humility
Negative aspects: Fear, Indecision, Willfulness, Mistrust

**Wood Element**
Liver and Gallbladder, SHHHHHHHHH
Spring
Green
Virtues: Generosity, Kindness, Patience, Clear thinking, Understanding
Negative aspects: Greed, Frustration, anger, impatience

**Fire Element**
Heart and Small Intestines, HAAAAAAAAAA
Summer
Red

Virtues: Joy, Happiness, Passion and Enthusiasm for life, honesty, respect, intuition

Negative aspects: Arrogance, rage, hatred, cruelty, haste

**Earth Element**

Stomach, Spleen, Pancreas, HOOOOOOOOOO (like the sound of a tiger)

Indian Summer

Yellow Gold

Virtues: Satisfaction, Fairness, Contentment, Balance, Support, Abundance

Negative aspects: Worry, Insecurity, Poor judgment, Anxiety

Endocrine Fire-Triple Warmer, HEEEEEEEEEEEE

Endocrine Glands: Pituitary, Pineal, Thyroid, Thymus, Pancreas, Adrenals, Ovaries and Testicles

Violet

Virtues: Effortless and Harmonious Communication, Creativity

Negative aspects: Imbalance, Miscommunication

# Bone Breathing Qigong

For thousands of years the Chinese have used various forms of Qigong exercise to realize better health. Bone Breathing is also referred to as iron shirt Qigong, due to it's association with the warrior monks (martial artists) in China and their use of this form to create a dense reservoir of chi in their bones, which established a strong layer of wei chi at the level of the skin.

Bone Breathing Qigong, a Taoist practice, is a practical way to increase the strength of the bones and the vitality of the blood. This active meditation is representative of the finest in Taoist Alchemy. With continued practice one may realize many benefits and positively shift blood enzymes to healthy levels; boosting immunity by bringing universal chi into the blood cells. Bones are relatively porous, and are therefore always "breathing." Bones are believed to vibrate like hollow reeds.

The effects of "Bone Breathing" Qigong are many. The practice prevents bone loss, reverses Osteoporosis, speeds healing, boosts the immune system, positively affects blood enzymes and increases your reserve of chi. After the chi gathers in the deepest part of the bone marrow it can expand out to the level of the skin. This creates a protective layer of chi, called "wei chi", which protects the body from invasion of negative chi and germs. Wei chi is what protects you when there is a change of weather, and the climate penetrates into the body creating damaging winds. Some references refer to this qigong form as Bone Marrow washing. Indeed the visualization and directing of chi through the bone marrow resembles a washing action. I like to imagine the ocean surf moving in and out of the bones.

The practice of bone breathing was introduced into the Western world by the Taoist teacher Mantak Chia in 1983. One of the first students was a middle aged woman residing in Los Angeles, California who was losing bone mass in her spine at an alarming rate. She was under the care of several specialists who had been unable to arrest the bone loss. The predicted outcome of her illness would be a spinal collapse threatening the nervous system and bringing paralysis or early death. As soon as she heard about bone breathing she enrolled in a class and began a daily routine of 3 hours of continuous exercise bringing subtle breath to the bone marrow. Since the skeleton is considered an antenna, the most efficient way of practicing bone breathing is standing up in a special posture that allows the complete skeleton to be aligned in the most efficient way with the flow of universal energies.

Within six months of practice she not only arrested bone mass loss but also began reversing the process and gained some 10% of the mass back. The doctors who had been treating her were at a loss to explain the reversal. Within three years of continued practice she began to appreciably regain bone mass and at the end of five years had replaced 100% her bone mass without indications that there had ever been osteoporosis.

This case is not an isolated one. Since the 1980's, similar cases have been reported by practitioners in different countries in Europe and the Americas. Bone breathing has been successfully used also for accelerated healing of broken bones and torn ligaments. An important condition in bone breathing practice is being able to feel the area being worked with the attention. The ancient Taoists have left us the maxim that says that "The practice of the Tao begins with feeling." Without feeling the practice may degenerate into being just a mental exercise unrelated to the bones." Juan Li from his website I Ching Dao.org

This type of Qigong would be considered Medical Qigong for its ability to improve health by bringing chi into the red and white blood cells in the bones. Red blood cells are formed in the long bones of the femur, humerus and tibia. White bloods cells form in the flat bones of the pelvis sternum and skull. When we are born our bones are heavy with circulation. Bones are associated with the water element, and Jing chi.

You are born with a natural amount of jing, and your lifestyle will affect how much energy, vitality and overall health you have each day. You can deplete your jing by indulging in too much of anything; food, sex, drugs, and unmanaged stress. Long term Stress and the production of Cortisol can promote bone loss, kidney damage, weight gain, immune system disorders, more.

As we enter menopause our body produces fewer hormones, such as estrogen and progesterone that maintain the health of our bones and the elasticity of our connective tissues. Possible consequences of this slowing down in hormone production can be osteoporosis and heart disease, wrinkled skin, lowered vitality and decreased libido. 8 to 10 times more women than men experience osteoporosis, (porous bones). Estrogen withdrawal after menopause is associated with a rapid and sustained increase in the rate at which bone is lost.

This phenomenon seems to result from an increase in bone resorption that is not met by an equivalent increase in bone formation. Osteoclasts out produce osteoblasts. Up to 20% of your bones are recycled every year. The 206 bones in your body are continually remodeling themselves.

As we age the bones become fatty and brittle, and bone marrow is less vibrant. Bone breathing qigong practice can prevent and reverse this thinning of the bones. It is a fine example of a Yang Shen, Longevity practice as well as a Healing and Curing practice.

**Bones** are a living tissue, constantly creating new bone cells and carrying away old bones cells. Osteoclasts carry away the old and osteoblasts stimulate the new.

*Think of your bones as a structural reservoir of essential life supporting minerals, like calcium and phosphorus.*

**Bone marrow** is the spongy tissue inside our bones. All bones in newborn babies have active marrow, which means they are producing new marrow cells. By the time a child reaches young adulthood, the marrow inside the bones of the hands, feet, arms, and legs stop producing new marrow cells. In adults, active marrow is found inside the spine, hip and shoulder bones, ribs, breastbone, and skull. However, bone marrow found in the spine and hip has the richest source of bone marrow cells.

Like many of our historical references, the personal stories of the success of Bone Breathing Qigong are anecdotal and not peer-reviewed scientific studies. However, the desired result will happen if one practices regularly with clear intention. I personally have felt a huge boost in my energy levels throughout the day when I have done Bone Breathing. And I have seen students with broken bones heal quickly using this practice when all other methods failed. A student of mine who practices acupuncture in New York found that her cancer patients experienced relief from neuropathy when they listened to the bone breathing qigong CD. This is a great example of a practice which enhances our immune system and shifts blood enzymes. Another student of mine shared this with her friend while he was in the hospital. After one session the hospital staff discovered inadvertently that his liver enzymes had changed for the better. And there are more success stories from around the world.

In Traditional Chinese Medicine the term marrow (Sui) is considered the substance that is the common matrix of bones, bone marrow, spinal cord and brain. Marrow circulates chi and irrigates the bones. The Chinese character for "Sui" is composed of the combination of images below. Bone on the upper left, flesh and tissues on the lower left, lower right image depicts the idea of building something and something walking aside the building. This represents the movement of marrow inside the bones. Marrow nourishes the bones, spinal cord and the brain.

This practice can be done standing, sitting or lying down. If you practice standing you become solidly grounded and strengthen your ability to direct chi through your skeletal system. The more grounded you are the more the chi rises up. If you are not feeling well, sitting is the best posture.

It is invigorating and a good practice to do on a daily basis, a practical and profound method of Medical Qigong. For both women and men Bone Breathing qigong is especially good for maintaining healthy marrow. Therefore it is included in both the curing and healing practices as well as the prevention and longevity practices.

**Breath, Visualization and Posture**
Using your breath and your ability to visualize is where this begins. If you are standing find a comfortable stance with soft knees. I like to begin by moving with my breath, sinking on the inhale and standing up and pushing my palms toward the earth on the exhale. This gentle up and down movement keeps me relaxed as I breathe a guide the chi into the bones. If you are sitting our laying down, begin by connecting with your breath in a focused way on the inhale and exhale. This does not have to be a really big breath, just a conscious breath.

*Open your chi field to the primordial chi field of infinite source. Connect with the highest, purest source of chi that you can imagine, and beyond.*

We enlist our ability to visualize, which may seem like simple a mental practice, yet it is one of our strongest allies in self-healing. Many Taoist practices seem to begin with a mental approach, but actually this gives the mind a job, allows you to focus, and eventually the mind gets out of the way. To affect healing, Chi needs guiding and purifying. What happens is that we gradually begin to FEEL the chi moving in the bones. Some chi sensations are pleasant, and some are not. If the chi has been blocked in an area on your bones, you may feel nothing, or you may feel warmth and tingling, or a jolting sensation.

Every one of us is different every time we practice. I was practicing Bone Breathing the day after I injured my leg and knee playing tennis. The chi shot through my leg like a lightning rod and straightened it out.

Now that you are connected to pure Universal Chi, bring your attention to the tips of your toes, all 10 toes, and imagine that there are openings like straws at the tips of all your toes. Invite pure chi to enter the small bones of your toes on the inhale, swirling, stimulating and clearing out the marrow. On the exhale release the old chi. Continue bringing in fresh chi and releasing old chi on each breath. Do this for several breaths before moving on. If you are doing this alone you may want to look at a picture of the skeleton before you begin to refresh your memory of the many bones in your body. There are approximately 200 bones.

You can imagine the chi as a color if this helps you to visualize. I picture the chi moving in and out like the waves coming in on a shoreline and retreating with the old chi. I enjoy this image as an example of bone marrow washing.

Continue breathing and visualizing the chi moving up the toes to the feet, ankles, legs, knees, femur, hips, pelvis, spine, and ribs. Take your time in each location and notice what you feel, or if there is a lack of feeling.

Now bring your attention to your fingertips; all 10 fingers. Breathe into the small bones of the fingers trying to imagine the shape of the bones and the bone marrow. Continue to the bones of the hands, wrists, forearms, elbows, humerus, shoulder, scapula, clavicle, head, jaw and teeth.

Now you are breathing into all of the bones of the body at once. Continue with a few more breaths and then rest. Notice how your body is moving through space. Notice if you feel more grounded and present. Are your bones feeling heavy?

After several months of this practice you can begin Bone Packing. I will cover this in another chapter that will lead you into the practice of Buddha Palms.

When one feels the resiliency of strong, supple bones and a cheerful vitality exuding from the blood, self-esteem improves and the quality of life experiences are enhanced to their fullest enjoyment.

*The Bone Breathing CD that I have recorded is beneficial in many ways. It is great for improving one's overall vitality, and is also very effective for those healing from diseases and chemotherapy because it can be done lying down. It improves the regeneration of bone marrow and bone strength, and strengthens the immune system.

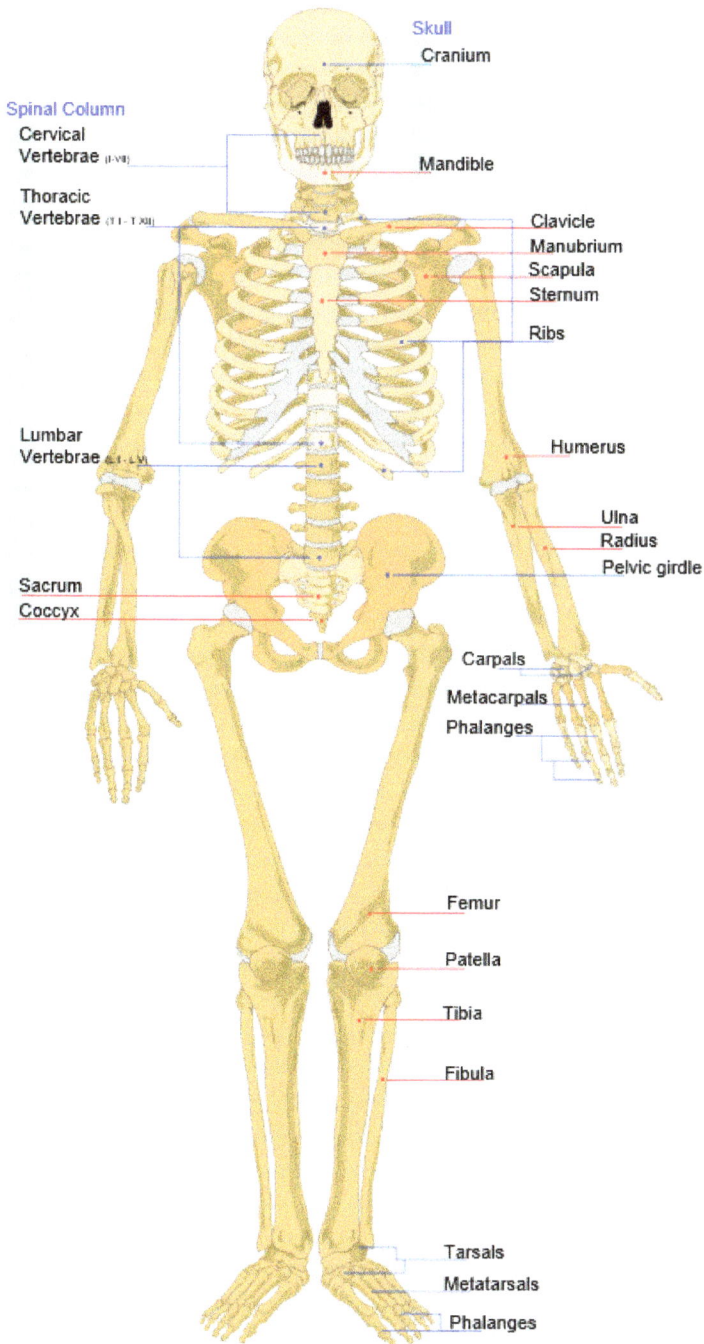

Skull
Cranium

Spinal Column
Cervical
Vertebrae (I-VII)

Mandible

Thoracic
Vertebrae (T I - T XII)

Clavicle
Manubrium
Scapula
Sternum

Ribs

Lumbar
Vertebrae (L I - L VI)

Humerus

Ulna
Radius
Pelvic girdle

Sacrum
Coccyx

Carpals
Metacarpals
Phalanges

Femur

Patella

Tibia

Fibula

Tarsals
Metatarsals
Phalanges

# Conscious Breathing

*"Regulate the breathing and harvest gold in a Cauldron"*

-Sun Buer

Breath and consciousness are intimately connected. 28,000 times every day our lungs and diaphragm move independently. If we pay attention to this automatic breathing we can trace the physical and emotional reality of our lives. And, if we focus our awareness on our breath, taking a more conscious breath with specific intentions and movements of the body, we affect our mind and body; the vagus nerve relaxes, diaphragmatic breathing moves lymph, strengthens heart rate variability, and slows brain waves. Daoist practitioners discovered that when the mind calms during meditation we shift from watching the breath to deep a stillness of the Void or Primordial Chi. Breathing keeps the balance of Yin and Yang, extracts negative ions from the air and alkalinizes the blood.

Sun Buer advises us to "keep the mind clear like water, and the heart still like a mountain. Regulate the breathing and harvest gold in a Cauldron." That cauldron is the lower tan tien which is contacted with deep breathing using the diaphragm.

The breathing pattern that is used in Daoist meditation is simple, natural and consistent throughout all practices from sitting meditation to standing qigong. Even the sexual practices use this method to circulate chi.

The pattern is this: Let the diaphragm drop and the pelvic floor relax on the inhale. Fill the lungs and let the ribs expand, feel the organs being massaged as the belly expands on the inhale. On the exhale pull up the pelvic floor, close the earthly gate, draw the diaphragm up and take a complete exhale. It is important to exhale completely and pause at the bottom of this exhale to allow the next inhale to come naturally.

This focused way of breathing will become second nature with practice. In her poems, Sun Buer mentions several times the breath as a way to accomplish internal alchemy.

Breathing as a medical therapy was recorded on jade tablets in the 6th century BC in China, and was highly recommended by Dr. Sun Simiao, a renowned physician.

*Respiration: re spiriting the body. As we breathe we refine the spirit into the world of matter. Count your life by the number of breaths you take.*

As a healing or curing practice Conscious Breathing is essential to bring fresh chi and oxygen into the body. It is recommended that we relax our eyes (simply un-focus them, no need to close them) and bring our focus inside several times a day to assist the liver to produce fresh blood and to carry off toxins. Stress creates an acidic environment in our body which fuels disease. Conscious breathing will quickly alkalinize the blood and bring us back to a relaxed state for healing.

Breathing will also allow us to keep track of our emotions. The lungs are representative of the Metal element. When we are strong in this element, we can acknowledge our emotions, let go of what is not needed, and find the courage to move forward. What we become aware of during conscious breathing will change with our inner observations and meditations. This is a simple law of physics; observation creates events. What we are not aware of can cause damage to our health. We often hold our breath to avoid feelings, and when we are concentrating the mind intently on a thing. This holding is not beneficial to the organs and to our overall health.

If you are lying down a lot due to illness, the lungs will become weak. Rest your hands on your lower belly and fill your lower abdomen on the inhale. Exhale completely, pressing your belly with your hands if necessary.

It is a good idea to sit up for short periods, if possible, and Breathe. There are many qigong forms that synchronize breath and movement. These movements guide the chi through meridians and focus the mind. When you are strong enough you may sit up and move your arms, reaching up, as you breathe. When you are even stronger, stand while you practice breathing exercises and include a few slow qigong arm movements.

According to the Daniel Reid, the nutrition provided by air through breathing is even more vital to health and longevity than that provided by food and water through digestion.

# Walking as a Medical Qigong Prescription

Walking to restore and preserve health is a classic medical Qigong prescription. I have met several walkers on the mountain paths in China, who proudly proclaimed their advanced age and how fit they were as walkers. Indeed, many of the mountain hermits rely on the ability of walkers carrying large heavy packages on bamboo poles up narrow mountain paths. Walking is the most natural movement for a human body, one learned in the first year of life. Forest Bathing from Japan is now coming to popular attention as a healing activity.

In Traditional Chinese Medicine, Walking is one of 4 classic prescriptions for treating cancer. The 4 are: Nutrition and Herbs, Deep Breathing Therapy, Walking, and Tone Resonation Therapy. In Ancient China Taoist Qigong walking training was divided into 3 modalities; 1. Eliminating illness and extending life 2. Returning all things to the root 3. Obtaining mastery of adaptation. Today in China medical qigong clinics focus primarily on walking techniques for eliminating illness and extending life. This type of walking therapy is most like Forest Bathing in concept. Eliminating illness and extending life strengthens the bodys's Jing and encourages the absorption of substances while walking. The Forest Bathing style of walking absorbs phytoncides from trees in the forest.

Shinrin-yoku is a term that means "taking in the forest atmosphere" or "forest bathing." It was developed in Japan during the 1980s and has become a cornerstone of preventive health care and healing in Japanese medicine. Researchers primarily in Japan and South Korea have established a robust body of scientific literature on the health benefits of spending time under the canopy of a living forest.

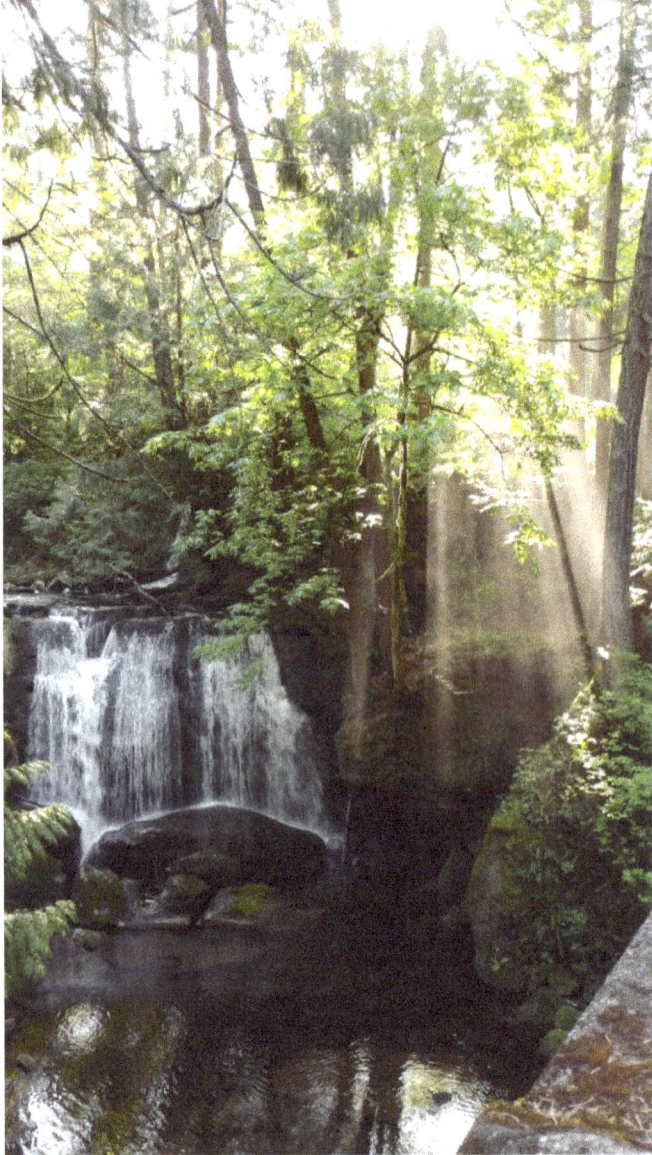

**What's in the Air?**

Under the canopy of Evergreen trees we are bathing in an atmosphere of phytoncide rich air. All plants have phytoncides: active substances with antimicrobial properties that kill or inhibit the growth of bacteria, fungi and protozoa. Cedars must be very good at this since nothing grows on them even when the dead logs are lying on the ground. Some trees release in to the atmosphere volatile phytoncides that are capable of producing an effect at a distance. Studies have shown that the air in coniferous forests, and particularly in young pine forests, is practically sterile and free of harmful microflora.

Forest Bathing and breathing in the fresh Chi of nature produces mental, emotional and physical healing, and more. Forest plants emit essential wood oils and airborne chemicals to protect themselves from insects and decay.

Studies show that forest aromas benefit humans as well. Forest bathing reduces stress and the stress hormone cortisol, lowers blood sugar, increases concentration, strengthens the immune system, builds up vitality, increases Heart Rate variability, elevates mood, decreases blood pressure, increases the levels of natural killer cells, and more.

All cultures recognize that trees uplift the human spirit. To ancient people, trees were channels for the gods; forests were human's first temples and sanctuaries. Japanese Shinto religion sees trees and all of nature as having indwelling spirits. The mountains of China are covered with paths leading to temples and tea houses.

**Walking like the Wind**

Inner stillness and outer movement must be harmonized in Walking therapy. From a Chinese medicine point of view Walking will stimulate the meridians of the feet and legs, increase blood and lymph flow, stimulate the appetite, strengthen the heart and lungs and provide a way to relax the mind and emotions. Each step is a focused meditation.

Both Chinese Qigong Walking therapy and Forest Bathing therapy have preparation and closing activities for the walker. Chinese Qigong Walking therapy uses the breath and arm movements to expel toxic chi by visualizing the internal organs and releasing this chi from the body. Imagine a dark chi exiting the body from all pores and being absorbed into the earth for re cycling. Find a movement of your arms that symbolizes releasing.

Daoist tree meditation connects one to a specific tree and circulates chi between oneself and the tree in a circle coming through the feet and the tree roots and back to the sky and crown of the head.

Preparation for Forest Bathing includes creating a specific intention to connect with nature in a healing way with mindfulness, presence, opening all the senses, and actively communicating. Communing with nature creates a relationship with nature. There is a still consciousness in nature that we are a part of, especially in trees. Forest bathing walks are of a short distance and slow paced.

The Wood element in Chinese medicine holds the superior virtues of patience and generosity. The breathing that happens while we walk frees up the Liver chi and enriches the blood. When Liver chi is fresh and clear we are able to think clearly. Making clear minded decisions is essential during a time of healing.

Fast and slow walking methods are prescribed for patients in the various stages of a disease. In the beginning you may only walk a very short distance for 5-10 minutes. As your stamina returns you may walk further, for up to 20 minutes. The focus of these walks is to strengthen and heal the body, not to accomplish any specific exercise goal.

Forest bathing recommends a "sit spot" during a walk. Find a sit spot, communicate, watch, listen, smell, touch, taste, intuit. Notice everything around you and inside of you; be curious. Your senses bring you into the present moment. Nature is our best teacher.

Chinese Medical Qigong Therapy closes a walking session by massaging the lower tan tien to bring the accumulated chi into the Jing level of the body. Self-massage is done after any Daoist meditation session and there are many ways to do this. Most commonly we massage the face, arms, legs and kidneys.

For more specific stepping and walking therapy prescriptions which include mudras, you might like to consult J. A. Johnson's Volume 2 of Chinese Medical Qigong Therapy.

# Qigong

Many of our beautiful flowing Qigong forms have been handed down from masters and today we are discovering how to balance our lives with some very simple, yet powerful meditative movements.

Qigong is moving meditation. Let's take a look at the word; Qigong. It is made up of two Chinese characters; Qi or Chi, meaning air, or a universal energy that permeates and flows thru everything; the breath that we all breathe, and Gong; which represents the effort or practice of learning to interact with chi and cultivate it for healing.

Qigong is a meditative practice of moving chi through the inside and around the outside of the body to affect balance and better health. Sometimes likened to fishing without a hook, qigong increases our awareness of our personal chi field and then we sense what is needed for balance.

The ancient Chinese sages or *Wu* created *Qigong* as a life science system to maintain the health of the body, mind, and spirit. It stems from classical Daoist traditions and is rooted in the principles of Classical Chinese Medicine.

In its true form, *Qigong* is a practice for cultivating knowledge and a main method for moving into *Tian Ren He Yi* (the state of oneness of the universe and the human being). *Qigong* is translated into English as '*Qi* cultivation' or 'to work with the *Qi*.' There are many forms of *Qigong* practice: sitting meditation, movement (including Taijiquan and other internal martial arts), breath work, regulation of mental focus and emotions, visualizations, mudras, and mantras.

The proper use of herbal supplements and food choices can be associated with Qigong. Cultivation of the classical arts -- such as calligraphy and music -- is considered a form of Qigong when conducted in a mindful manner.

In any case, all the different forms have the same three keys, or three alignments: regulating the posture, regulating the breath, and regulating the mind. "Qigong facilitates the development of a deeper relationship with Qi. This relationship helps the practitioner understand the laws of the universe and how they influence human life." Master Zhongxian Wu, Vital Breath of the Dao, page 78.

There are thousands of Qigong forms, many developed specifically by individuals over the past centuries to heal specific ailments. If you are healing at this time in your life, choose a simple form of Qigong that does not tire you, but allows you to feel refreshed and energized.

There are Martial forms of Qigong like Bone Breathing, or Bone Marrow Washing and Tan Tien Qigong which come from the Iron Shirt Tradition. There are Spiritual forms of Qigong like Primordial Qigong and Dream practices. The Alchemical branch of Qigong includes meditations such as the Inner Smile and 6 Healings Sounds, Microcosmic Orbit, and Fusion of the 5 Elements. And there are Medical Qigong forms, like the ones I learned at the Xi Yuan hospital in Bejing which balance the organs energy. And there are specific forms to strengthen blood flow and the Liver, like Jade Woman.

Many Qigong forms include slow meditative movements, yet the most advanced forms do not require physical movement, only the directing of the chi through the organs and meridians of the body, to affect balance of chi flow for optimum health.

Chi takes on many qualities. It can be vibrant and of high quality or stagnant and charged with low level energy. We individually live with chi that is either enlivening and in balance, or weak and disease producing, in excess or deficient. With conscious practice, observation and quiet reflection we can learn to evaluate and work with our chi level and how it flows through our bodies. The quality and quantity of chi can change moment to moment. It is our opportunity to affect our post heavenly chi in these moments.

We gather chi from the air, food, water, nature, and from sleeping. Our thoughts and emotions affect the quality and quantity of chi. Qigong practice teaches us to feel, sense, purify, cultivate, circulate, store and project chi for healing. As we become still we become more attuned to where we are out of flow, or out of balance. This awareness then allows us to restore harmony and balance.

As we move gently with Qigong, the breathing becomes deeper and the mind quiets. The blood shifts back into a more balanced ph which allows for deeper meditation. Life events and emotions become less intense as the body and its glands and organs find new balance and fill with the higher virtues that we were born with.

With simple and consistent practice we begin to cultivate life, and return our energy to pure source and the realm of primordial awareness.

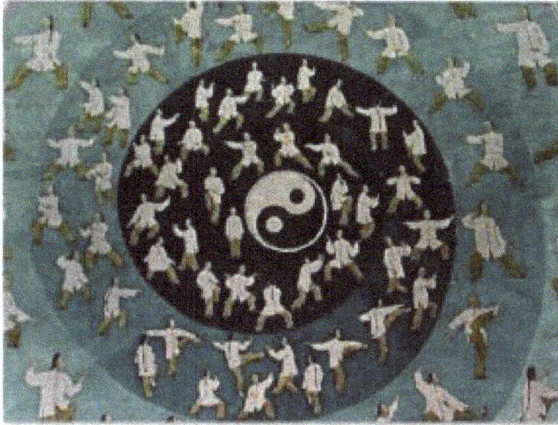

**How do Seasonal Qigong Forms support your health and vitality?**

Humans are Nature. Our rhythms move naturally with the movement of the sun, moon, (light and dark) planets and stars, tides and rivers, the flowering and fruiting of plants, the movement of animals and birds. Even the digestion of our foods is dependent on what is available each season. Everything that we need to know about our world and keeping healthy can be found simply or metaphorically in nature.

Our breath is just right for a human body. The respiration of a tree is just right for the tree. Both have consciousness and ways of communicating. The planet has one breath each year, an inhale and an exhale. Drawing in chi and letting go of chi as the earth moves on its axis. The hummingbird has a quick movement, the galaxies a much slower movement.

Qigong movements create a flow of chi through the body and its structure; the meridians. Each meridian is a river of chi moving between the interior and the exterior of the body, from organs to the extremities and back. Every organ has it's season, sound, and color, and time of day. And therefore we can use qigong to strengthen the organs and our overall health by choosing a movement which recognizes the organ and brings more chi into the organ. Sound and color produce a quality of chi. Movement creates a flow of chi.

For example, during the Spring it is a great idea to choose movements that clear and tonify the Liver chi. Locate the liver and gallbladder meridians and make some movements, or do some stretches and massage for the liver and gallbladder meridians. Make it fun. And send some vibrant spring green color from your mind's eye into the liver and gallbladder to tonify them. Sounds will break up stagnation and move out stuck chi. Try the sound Shhhhh and see the old chi moving out of your liver to be recycled by the universe.

Each Season/Element has a movement. Winter/Water brings us to a still point; a place of rest and rejuvenation. When we give ourselves the gift of stillness our entire being has an opportunity to become refreshed. Winter Qigong forms that I teach focus on slow movements to open the kidney and bladder meridians, and have longer quiet sitting meditations. I allow the natural darkness to fill the room. Pearl of the Night is a Winter Qigong form that I created. It is very simple and restorative.

Spring/Wood begins the movement upward and outward like the sap rising in the trees, stimulated by the wind moving the woods. Traditionally we use this time of year to detoxify our bodies. Nature, and our liver, is pushing chi up and out through branches and meridians. Qigong forms that stimulate the liver are great for Spring. I like forms like Swimming Dragon which open the spine and Jade Woman which clears liver chi.

Spontaneous Qigong might look like a dance, or child's play. Let yourself move randomly, or shake. Let your breath and movement be natural and easy.

There are many forms to choose from, so begin with something that you like and continue to practice with an easy open mind and body. I like to do a short Qigong warmup sequence before I decide what specific form I want to do. I may focus on one "form" for a season or a place that I am in. Some movements are common to many forms, and although they are the same movement they have different names.

One of these is a simple movement that is done from a standing posture with the arms at the sides of the body. Turn your palms to face the sky and raise both arms up, as if you are gathering heavenly chi. When you reach to top of your head, bring your hands down through your central channel toward the earth. Continue this circular movement for several minutes and sense the changes that it creates.

Ask yourself how the movement feels to you; does it challenge you or does it calm you? I ask that my Qigong teachers in training keep a journal of their qigong practice experiences.

My recommendation is that you find a class, a local instructor, a Qigong DVD, or a book that appeals to you and begin with some simple movements. Trust your experience and continue to learn how to care for yourself.

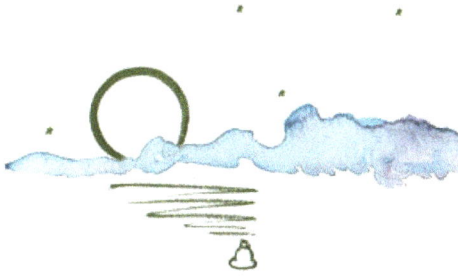

# Meditation

Meditation is a form of qigong for the mind. The physical body needs to be developed and prepared as a tuning fork for meditation. Qigong is a highly adaptable and pleasant way to prepare. Many Daoist meditations result in creating a positive alchemical change in the physical body which leads to better health and emotional balance, and providing a clear channel for spiritual awareness. The true purpose is to align our microcosm (body) with the macrocosm (universe) and to be one with all Nature and the infinite Chi field which is life and universal, infinite space. The space within mirrors the space without; as above, so below.

The classic Daoist way of meditation is called 'sitting in oblivion'; doing nothing but allowing everything to be done. The symbol, or trigram, for meditation is the mountain which represents stillness. Hexagram #52 of the I Ching is mountain over mountain, (mountain doubled) or keeping still. When you sit in meditation you take on the posture of a still mountain. Sun Bu'er advises the Daoist practitioner; "The mind needs to be clear, like water, the heart needs to be still, like a mountain".

We affect the quality and quantity of chi in many ways; the air we breathe, the food we eat, the emotions we feel, our thoughts, our posture, the water we drink, the environment we are in, our sexual behavior, sleeping, exercise, etc..... In order to be successful in meditation practice we must have a good quantity and quality of chi to move within the body. And so our daily activities and choices affect our meditation and spiritual practice. We can cultivate chi daily in all of the ways mentioned here, and we can also conserve chi when it is necessary for healing.

There are 4 steps to bring us into meditation; Relaxation (surrender), Concentration on the lower tan tien, Focus (in spite of distractions remain focused), and Levitation (the burden of life is shed and you experience a new reality or an awareness outside of the usual orientation of time and space in daily living).

There is no time limit in the spiritual world, you may experience a gradual or a spontaneous process, and should never compare yourself to others, yet have perseverance. Given the right time or place you will reach a sensation to examine something, to look inside yourself. Your meditation time needs to include some preparation of the physical space so that you are not disturbed or interrupted. When we meditate, the parts of our brain which orients us in time and space go quiet; we therefore, lose track of time and space, even feeling expansion and lightness of being. This is called "zero point."

The best time for gathering and cultivating chi is between the hours of dawn until midday as the yang energy is rising.

During the afternoon and evening, Yin energy returns, and therefore this is the best time for practicing tao yin and fertility practices.

If you like Incense chose a pine fragrance, as this opens the lungs and allows you to breathe deeply and moves awareness to the heavens like a tall pine tree.

Color opens consciousness and it is acceptable to imagine chi having a color as you guide it in the body. Sound purges stagnation and opens the pathway for chi to move. Some sounds and mantras are helpful, like the Six Healing Sounds.

Sitting is the most common meditation posture. Find a comfortable sitting position with your spine straight. Standing is more demanding, but works well in many cases, as in bone breathing. Lying down is the most difficult posture for maintaining focus, one might fall asleep and the chi may pool in the chest or head, however, if you are ill then lying down is acceptable. When you want to complete your meditation, return your radiant pearl of chi to the lower tan tien; into the cauldron.

I teach a meditation called the 9 turns, which is a sleeping meditation, and it is done lying down. The practitioner guides the chi around the body through several meridians to slow the chi and relax the body. This meditation begins and ends at the navel. Daoist Dream Practice is also done lying down. In Dream Practice we are using sleep to activate consciousness. Meditation is a conscious form of sleep.

The Daoist point of view is that the body is as important as the mind. Reality tells us that we have a physical body which allows us to experience life on Earth.

*The highest form of medicine is prevention. Daily meditation practice brings daily awareness, balance and harmony to the heart/mind and spirit. What you become aware of you may affect. Observation changes events.*

Meditation practice will refine your chi and bring new awareness. With this refined chi you can utilize the awareness and the surplus of chi to support your state of equilibrium and healing.

Don't have an expectation of what should happen, simply participate in your life. Go fishing without a hook. Ask yourself, "what is right with me and my life." Don't criticize yourself and look for faults. Support your life and your healing with positive thoughts and experiences.

Previous chapters in this manual discuss the Inner Smile and 6 Healing Sounds, Bone Breathing, and Qigong as a moving meditation. These are good daily meditations. Walking can become a meditation practice.

Deep contemplation of nature is one form of meditation; extending your vision and chi field out to merge with Nature, and then bringing that awareness back into your personal landscape. If you are outside and can see the horizon, allow your eyes to travel to the furthest horizon, and expand your chi field. Then bring your vision back into your immediate surroundings, thereby concentrating your chi near to your body.

I will introduce you to a very simple meditation practice here. Choose a time and place that is conducive to mediation, where you will not be interrupted for at least 45 minutes. Sit cross legged, if possible, with your open palms resting on your thighs. If you cannot sit with legs crossed you can sit in a chair with your hands resting below your navel. Women will place the left hand on top of the right hand as it covers the lower tan tien. Bring your attention to the breath, making no noise as the air comes and goes from the nose. Focus on the lower abdomen, and feel the movement of your diaphragm as you inhale and exhale. Feel your ribs expanding on the inhale, and pull up the pelvic floor on the exhale. This pulling up, or closing of the earthly gate on the exhale, nourishes the internal organs of the pelvis. Keep your inhale and exhale slow, steady and even. Breathe as if you are spinning silk. Feel the movement of your internal universe.

When you are finished with your sitting meditation, move gently and slowly. Massage along the arms and legs to encourage chi to flow in the meridians. Cover your eyes with your hands, relaxing them from the internal viewing. Massage your face and ears.

# Chi Nei Tsang

## Self care
*Abdominal Massage to improve digestion and elimination*

Chi Nei Tsang literally translates to bring chi into the internal organs. CNT abdominal massage is one of the four branches of Traditional Chinese Medicine; Massage, Herbs, Acupuncture and Qigong. This healing practice is very old and probably pre dates Acupuncture as a healing modality.

Chi Nei Tsang is taught to massage therapists and other hands on therapists, however, the following self-care routine is taught to them as well. We can take responsibility for our health with this technique. Be gentle, and be curious. Get to know your own belly, don't inflict pain and you will not hurt yourself. If you discover an area that is frequently tender, seek out the advice of a professional. Visceral restrictions and adhesions cause limited motion in the organs, and also affect the spine and posture. You may work on yourself daily.

If you are lying down or sitting most of the day because you have been ill, then it is very beneficial to do Chi Nei Tsang breathing as this moves lymph and blood in the belly and assists the organs metabolism.

**Self Care Routine**
1. Lie down on your back in a comfortable, quiet place. Bend your knees so that your back is relaxed and your feet are flat on the floor. Put a few pillows under your knees to support them in this relaxed position.

2. Place your hands on your belly and breathe deeply, filing your abdomen first and then let the breath rise up into your lungs. Exhale completely and wait until the next breath comes naturally. Notice any places that hesitate to take in breath and chi. Observe any emotion that arises with the breath. Continue breathing with conscious awareness for several minutes.

3. Use your fingers to feel the texture of the skin inside the rim of your navel. Massage firmly in all directions inside the navel to about 1/2 of the depth of your navel. Allow time for the navel to shift and change; it is connected to all parts of your body via the connective tissue. Feel the energetic connections from your navel to other places in your body. You may use various methods of massage, (circles, pulsing, or simply holding a stretch). Take as much time as you need, this may become a large segment of the self-care massage.

4. Move your hands to the lower left quadrant of the abdomen and find the sigmoid and descending colon. Gently pump the large intestine with your fingers. This creates circulation, hydration, intestinal transit and affects the movement of lymph of the pelvis.

5. Continue this technique along the entire length of the descending colon, transverse colon and ascending colon, ending at the cecum in the lower right quadrant of the abdomen. At the flexures of the intestine, under the rib cage on right and left sides, stretch the tissues down to create more space for the breath to move the diaphragm. If there is pain anywhere, pause and breathe, allowing the tissues to respond.

6. Create small circles on your belly with your fingers above the small intestine, moving in larger spirals out from the navel until you have felt the entire area of the small intestine.

7. Explore areas of your belly that call out to you for attention and relaxation; (if you have consistent complaints from your stomach, small intestine, liver and gallbladder, or anywhere else, then spend some time with your hands to massage gently and send healing chi and a smile into the area.

8. Rest and return to your breath. Notice the changes that have occurred in your belly and your awareness. Smile.

# Acupressure for Self Care

*Enlivening the Immune System*

Acupressure predates Acupuncture however both practices utilize the same points along meridians to regulate the chi that flows through the body. Acupressure uses firm, gentle pressure with one's fingers rather than needles. A 10-15 minute self-care treatment can strengthen a weak immune system and restore a sense of wellness. 5000 years ago the Chinese discovered that certain points on the body relieved pain where it was felt, and also brought about a sense of relief in distant areas of the body. Meridians connect all of the points on each meridian pathway to a specific organ, which is what causes the distant relief.

This science developed by trial and error over many years of observation. Stimulating acupressure points triggers a release of endorphins; neurochemicals, which relieve pain. Pain and tension seem to gather around points that are stagnated, which makes finding them easier.

There are twelve meridians that move chi between our organs and our extremities and they follow a specific pathway and time table every day. (See the timetable of the meridians graph on page 17) Eleven meridians flow to and from organs and the twelfth meridian is called the Triple Warmer, which balances all of the organs.

There are 365 common acupressure points, and each of these points have been given poetic names that evoke the action of the point. You can meditate on these names as you press and stimulate the points. For instance; CV (conception vessel) #17 is called the Sea of Tranquility, or Milk Flow. It is located on the sternum, 3 thumb widths up from the base of the sternum. The name for this point suggests a lovely focus for meditation as you touch the point, especially for Women. As chi gathers in this point you may notice that the thrusting channels (part of the 8 extraordinary vessels) that flow through breast tissue begin to fill and bring sensation.

I have chosen 10 points for you to explore, as this section of the Women's Manual is about Curing and Healing, these 10 acupressure points will assist you to heal more quickly. You will want to find a good acupuncture or acupressure chart or book to assist with locating the points. My favorite book is "A Practical guide to Acu-points" by Jarmey and Bouratinos.

**Technique**
To release, sedate or reduce stuck chi in a point circle your finger in a counter clockwise rotation. When chi is stuck in a point there may be pain and tenderness there as you press. The point may also feel thick or dense. Think of a dam in a river which is blocking the flow of water. To tonify and bring chi into a point, circle your finger in a clockwise rotation. A point that needs tonifying may feel empty or vacant to your touch. At all times be gentle. Set your intention to create ease of flow and harmony in your body.

Find a comfortable private place where you will not be interrupted for 30-45 minutes.

**Points to palpate for this immune boosting treatment:**

*Bladder 23 and 47* are on the back near your waist to the sides of the spine, between L2 and L3. Use your fists to massage up and down on both points at the same time. "Sea of Vitality"

*Kidney 27* is below the clavicles near the sternum. "Elegant Mansion"

*Conception Vessel 17* on the sternum 3 thumb widths up from base of the sternum. "Sea of Tranquility" or "Milk Flow".

*Conception Vessel 6* is 2 fingers below the navel. "Sea of Energy"

*Stomach 36* is to the outside of the shin in the depression between bones. "Three Mile Point"

*Liver 3* is on the top of the foot in the valley between the big toe and second toe. "Bigger Rushing"

*Kidney 3* (not to be used after the first trimester of pregnancy) is found between the ankle bone and the Achilles tendon. "Bigger Stream"

*Triple Warmer 5* is two and one half finger widths above the crease in the wrist on the outside of the forearm. "Outer Gate"

*Large Intestine 11* is just above the elbow crease, outside arm. "Crooked Pond"

Take a few minutes after your self-care treatment to close your eyes and visualize the chi flowing smoothly through your body along the meridians, nourishing the organs and cells, bringing new vitality to your being.

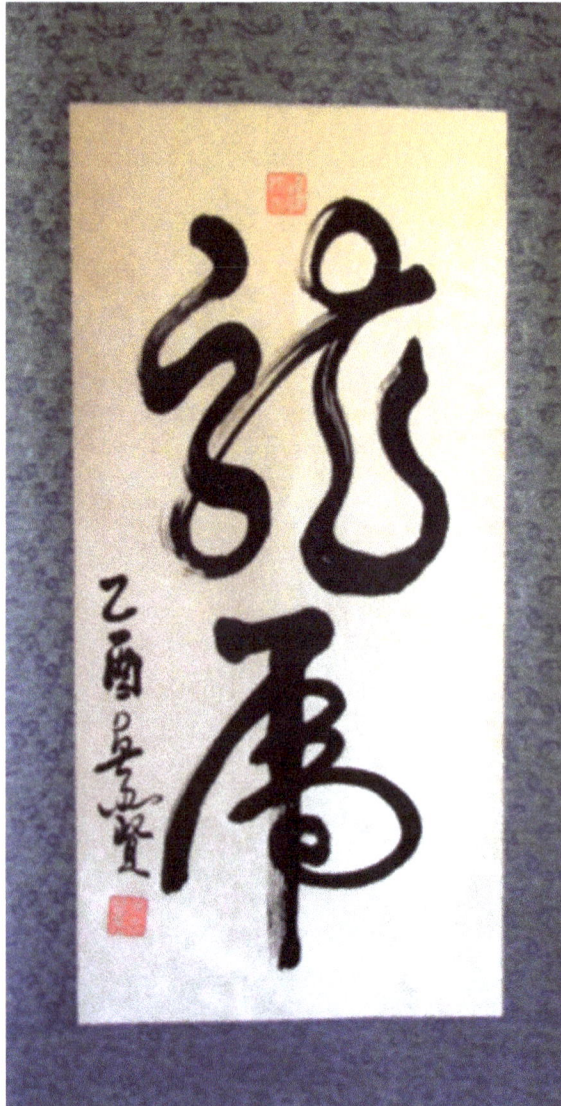

Dragon and Tiger calligraphy by Master Zhongxian Wu

# Mudras

## or Hand Seals "Shoujue"

Mudras created with fingers touching each other were used by Daoist Qigong masters. Specific hand postures are used to form a symbol with creates an energetic transformation and assists in healing diseases. Hand postures; Mudras, are designed to stimulate and increase the body's physical and spiritual potential, and are utilized with focus of mind, posture and breath, similar to Qigong practice.

Mudras are based upon the use of Yin and Yang energies. Using both hands will allow one to direct intention toward one goal. In ancient China, Daoist mystics would use the trigrams to summon the powers of specific elements, connecting the fingers in various patterns found in the Bagua. The Pure Yang Mudra explained here is an example of this type of mudra.

There are eight trigrams (patterns) formed by using Yin and Yang lines. They are Heaven, Earth, Fire, Water, Thunder, Mountain, Wind (or wood) and Lake. Four are Yin and four are Yang. Yin lines are broken and represent the number 6, Yang lines are solid and represent the number 9.

Qigong is much more than a technique for cultivation; it is the essence of ancient Chinese culture. Most people are unaware of the qi flowing through and around their bodies. Fortunately, this consciousness can be cultivated through specific Qigong practices. We can better understand what qi is and how it is connected with Chinese culture if we experience it through correct classical Qigong practice. Even in modern society, the majority of Qigong practitioners understand that practicing classical methods enhances personal abilities and benefits overall health.

One of the essential practices of classical Chinese Qigong is the Mudra. A mudra is a specific ritual common to ancient shamanism. In the Mt. Emei Sage Style Qigong (Emei Zhengong), we still preserve and utilize many special mudras as specific techniques of cultivation and healing/self-healing. The classical mudras, as representative of ancient symbols, carry and transmit ancient knowledge to us. The mudra has a deep relationship to one of the oldest records of ancient Chinese civilization, the *Book of Changes* (*Yijing*). In this context, it is more accurately translated as the *Classic of Symbols*.

Since the *Book of Changes* (*I Ching*) is considered the root of classical Chinese knowledge, science, and civilization, it can also be used to gain deeper insights into the foundation of Qigong theory. The symbolic meaning of a mudra may be understood by applying the symbolic knowledge first presented in the *Book of Changes*. As an ancient life science, Classical Chinese Medicine (CCM) is affiliated with both *Yijing* science and Qigong. Thus, mudras can also be understood through CCM theory." Master Zhongxian Wu, Empty Vessel Magazine, 2003.

Here are the meanings of the fingers from the Chinese tradition.

*Thumb* connects us to the outer world. It connects to the lungs and letting go.

*Index finger* indicates order in our lives.
Holding the mudra, index to thumb, advances our ability to let go of external concepts of order and control, to trust the universe and it's natural laws.

*Middle finger* is pericardium, which shields us and protects our heart

*Ring finger* is associated with the triple burner. For health 4$^{th}$ finger is most important. Touching the ring finger to the thumb will tonify liver and spleen.

*Pinky* finger relates to the heart and small intestine. The fire element represents control over one's life and Intuition.

You may create a mudra that fits your needs, and meditate on the symbolism.

**Pure Yang Mudra**
The Chinese name of Pure Yang Mudra is also a special symbol. In classical Chinese traditions, the function of a name is to carry and convey meaning in the same way a symbol carries and conveys complex levels of meaning. Therefore, the name of an object should carry all the information contained in that object.

The Chinese name of Pure Yang Mudra is "Chunyangyin", and this name carries multiple layers of meaning and contains its intentions. The original meaning of "Chun" is *silk* according to the second century dictionary, *Analyzing Simple Lines and Explaining Complex Graphs (Shuowen Jiezi)*. The symbolic meaning of "silk" is *white, pure,* and *linking/connecting*. Therefore, the character "Chun" exemplifies *pure, purity,* or *purifying*.

"Yang" contains many layers of meaning, including *sun, heaven, brightness, and south of a hill or north of a river*. "Yin" carries the meaning of *official seal*. In the terminology of the Daoist tradition, "yin" means *mudra*. Put together, these three terms make "Chunyangyin", which tells us that the function of this mudra is to help the practitioner connect with universal qi.

*This practice purifies the body and transforms the practitioner's energy into pure yang energy. Practicing the Pure Yang Mudra can enlighten the heart and the mind.*

Pure Yang energy is what is needed for healing and long life, it is not symbolic of becoming pure masculine. Understanding the background of the mudra through Mt. Emei Sage Style Qigong helps us grasp the deeper symbolic meanings of the Pure Yang Mudra.

Confucianism and Daoism, the two main pillars of classical Chinese tradition, both originated in the ancient world of shamanism. As the way of humanity, Confucianism inherited and rationalized the knowledge of courtesy, ceremonial rites and regulations, and aspects of personal emotion from the ancient shamanic rituals. As the way of nature, Daoism rationalized and expanded the wisdom of the universal way and applied pragmatic knowledge from the ancient shamanic rituals.

Pure Yang mudra is made by using both hands to form a ball with the little fingers, middle fingers, and thumbs softly touching, while the ring and index fingers remain open.

By carefully examining the formation of the Pure Yang Mudra, we can see that it has roots in the *Book of Changes*. The *Book of Changes* contains 64 hexagrams. A hexagram is constructed of six lines, three on the top and three on the bottom. Each set of three lines is called a trigram. To make a mudra the fingers come together to form the two trigrams that make up the hexagram.

You will see how the fingers form the two trigrams and resulting hexagram. Three fingers form the lower trigram: the little fingers connect, forming a yang line, the initial line; the ring fingers are open, forming a yin line, the second line; and the middle fingers connect, forming a yang line, the third line. This trigram is called "Li"; Fire.

The remaining 2 fingers form the upper trigram: the index fingers are open, forming a yin line, the fourth line; the thumbs connect, forming a yang line, the fifth line; and the sixth fingers, which form the sixth line, are nonexistent. Where is this sixth line? This line of the hexagram is hidden and cannot be seen. This trigram is called "Kan"; Water.

The two trigrams, "Kan" above and "Li" below, form hexagram #63 in the I Ching; *Book of Changes*. This is very symbolic; it is the fulfillment or completion. The last hexagram #64 is the beginning of a new cycle. #63 is the most perfect and balanced of all hexagrams.

Pure Yang Mudra creates the perfect alchemy of Fire and Water. As you hold this Mudra feel the Fire beneath the cauldron in your lower Tan Tien gently steaming your meridians and organs. Keep your breath deep and even to fan the fire. This is internal alchemy.

# Soups and Congee

Eating nutritious soups that are easy to digest is recommended when you are healing, or simply wanting to rest your body from any excess.

**7 Vegetables Soup**
This recipe was given to me by a friend from France. It came from his great grandmother who was the witch doctor in her native village in Southern Provence. It is recommended during any healing or cleansing times. This soup is simple, safe and inexpensive. When eaten on a regular basis it cleanses the digestive system of all excess. It is particularly good for the kidneys and liver. Eat this soup whenever you are sick or recovering from illness.

**Recipe**
Amounts for 1 person:
1 leek
1 turnip
1 carrot or 1 parsnip
1 small potato
1 small leafy green, such as chard or mustard greens (no cabbage, spinach or broccoli)
3 stalks celery
1 bunch parsley
Garlic (optional)
Seaweed (optional)

Rinse, dice and cover all of the vegetables in 1 quart of water. Add salt to taste. Cook until the carrots are tender. You may add chicken or an egg to the soup to make a full meal. I like to add Braggs' liquid aminos and miso.

## Bone Broth

Making bone broth is a potent way to bring deep healing chi into the body. Find organic beef or chicken bones at your grocery store and cook them overnight in a crock pot. Drink the broth plain, or add it to soups.

## Congee

A thin rice soup, with many health benefits. It is easy to digest and assimilate, strengthens the vitality and blood, balances the digestive organs, and promotes urination. It can be prepared with a variety of different herbal or food ingredients.

To prepare congee, use one part rice (white basmati works well), to five or six parts water. Simmer on low heat two to six hours. Stir occasionally. Crockpots work well.

For people who are very weak or seriously ill, or for supplementing mother's milk, the liquid can be strained off from the gruel, and taken alone.

Variations and additions to a basic rice Congee:

*Wheat congee:* cooling, calming, sedating.
*Sweet rice congee:* strengthening to the digestive organs and chi; good for vomiting and indigestion.
*Mung bean congee:* cooling.
*Aduki bean congee:* removes dampness, good for edema, gout, retention of urine and other kidney and bladder problems.
*Water chestnut congee:* cooling.

*Carrot congee:* carminative, good for indigestion and chronic dysentery.

*Spinach congee:* harmonizes and moistens organs.

*Celery congee:* cooling and relaxing to the liver.

Leek congee: warming and strengthening, good for chronic diarrhea.

*Pinenut congee:* moistens heart and lungs, harmonizes large intestine, good for constipation.

*Ginger congee:* warms cold digestive problems, such as vomiting, indigestion.

*Fennel congee:* carminative.

Other delicious and nutritious congees:
*Milk and honey congee.*
*Date, ginger, walnut, and honey congee.*

Chinese medicine uses numerous herbs in congee:
Wild yam, astragalus, asparagus, codonopsis, leichi berries, jujube, dong quai, longan fruit, ginseng.

## Kichari

Half and half basmati rice and mung beans, prepared as congee. This is considered to be the finest nutritive and detox food in Ayurveda. It is given during cleansing treatments, and after yogic purification. It is excellent as a mono diet for a week, with ghee, to cleanse the intestinal system, increase assimilation, and as part of an elimination diet to determine the causes of food reactions.

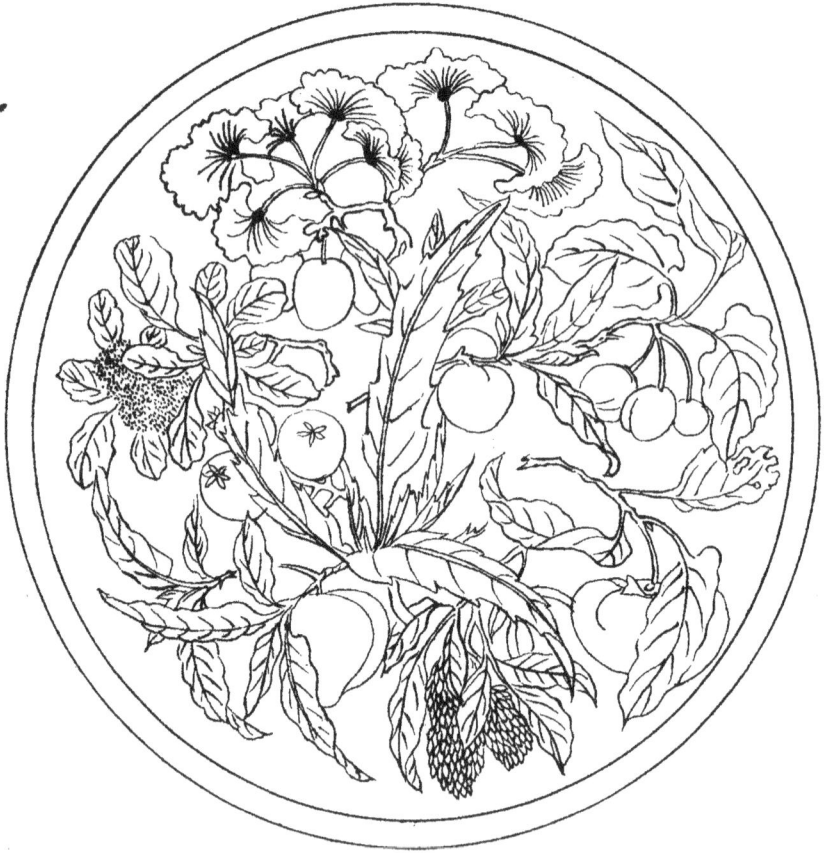

## SECTION 2

# YangSheng: Longevity & Prevention

## *Yangsheng* 养生 *(nourishing life)*

Yangsheng invites us to cherish life. It is best to restrain our desires for external things such as fame, fortune and power in order to nourish life. This includes the health of body, mind and emotions. Maintaining a peaceful mind and harmonizing the emotions are basic elements of longevity. Daoist practitioners who are nourishing life maintain a peaceful environment which is in harmony with nature. In this way one prevents imbalances which will bring harm to the life force. Longevity practices includes a variety of cultivation techniques, such as moderation in eating, meditation and breathing, exercises such as qigong and tai chi, Chi Nei Tsang, Bone breathing qigong, and Daoist sexual practices.

Once you have regained your health you can continue to incorporate those healing and curing practices into your Yangsheng practices, and add some new cultivation techniques which will further your physical foundation. When the body is at peace we can find the stillness of mind in our meditation.

# Bone Health

Bones are associated with the water element, and Jing chi. You are born with a natural amount of jing, and your lifestyle will affect how much energy, vitality and overall health you have each day. You can deplete your jing chi by indulging in too much of anything; food, sex, drugs, and unmanaged stress. Long term **Stress** and the production of Cortisol can promote bone loss, kidney damage, weight gain, immune system disorders, more.

As we enter menopause our body produces fewer hormones, such as estrogen and progesterone that maintain the health of our bones and the elasticity of our connective tissues. Possible consequences of this slowing down in hormone production can be osteoporosis and heart disease, wrinkled skin, lowered vitality and decreased libido. Eight to ten times more women than men experience osteoporosis (porous bones). Estrogen withdrawal after menopause is associated with a rapid and sustained increase in the rate at which bone is lost. This phenomenon seems to result from an increase in bone resorption that is not met by an equivalent increase in bone formation; osteoclasts out produce osteoblasts. Up to 20% of your bones are recycled every year. The 206 bones in your body are continually remodeling themselves.

Diet, lifestyle changes, qigong, meditation and herbs can prevent bone loss. Restoring Jing essence is a slow and deliberate process. **Digestion** is important to overall health, if you cannot absorb nutrients your bone health will suffer along with the rest of your body. It has been noted in the medical specialty of osteoimmunology that there is a correlation to gut problems like ulcerative colitis, Crohn's disease and bone loss. A healthy gut supports healthy bones; the large intestine produces some Vitamin K from the bacteria that live in it.

- Foods to include in your diet are dark leafy greens (**vitamin K**), beans, foods rich in **calcium**, zinc, copper, **vitamin D** and other minerals. Fish, nuts, seeds, olives and the oils that are produced from these foods are beneficial to bone health. Orange juice is high in calcium and vitamin D. Vitamin K is found in many fruits and vegetables; Kiwifruit, avocado, broccoli, green grapes, lettuce, parsley, prunes, kale, spinach, turnip greens, collards, parsley, romaine, green leaf lettuce, Brussels sprouts, cauliflower, cabbage, blackberries, figs, rhubarb can help you get your daily dose of this neglected nutrient. also oils (canola, soybean, and olive oil)

Vitamin K is a fat-soluble vitamin first identified in a study on blood coagulation by Carl Peter Henrik in Denmark. The letter "K" stands for "Koagulation", a Danish word for coagulation. Vitamin K is significantly at play in a wide range of biological activities including regulation of calcium metabolism in tissues, cell growth and proliferation, oxidative stress, inflammatory reactions, and blood coagulation and hemostasis.

Although vitamin K is not as significant to bone health as are calcium and vitamin D, low levels of circulating vitamin K have been linked with low bone density. Several studies have shown that supplementation with vitamin K results in improvements in bone health. In fact, new evidence points towards the potential role of this vitamin in:

- Slowing down bone loss after menopause in women
- Increasing bone strength and decreasing and/or limiting the risk of fractures in people suffering from osteoporosis

Support your health by reducing your intake of meats, dairy, caffeine and sugar. Cow's milk is high in protein, which creates acidity in the blood and causes the body to draw calcium from the bones to rebalance the ph in the body. One of my students who is a vegetarian was supplementing her diet with lots of cheese to meet her need for protein. She now has advanced Osteoporosis. While she was practicing Bone Breathing Qigong her bones rebounded, but since she stopped regular Qigong practice and began eating more cheese, she has lost ground.

Other ways to protect your bones are to avoid plastics with PCB which mimic estrogen. Soft drinks contain phosphoric acid which depletes the calcium in your bones. I know women who drink a diet coke every day and needed hip replacement when they were 60 due to pain and bone loss.

Heavy metals can build up in the bones, especially lead which seems to mimic calcium. If you are concerned about heavy metals please seek out a health care provider who can do test your levels and research ways to eliminate them from your body.

**Sunlight** is necessary to produce Vitamin D. In the past, Chinese women have sunbathed indoors through then rice paper screens that filtered out damaging UV rays, but allowed beneficial rays to reach the body.

Stimulate your bones with simple **exercises**, like walking or qigong and tai chi. 20 minutes 3 or 4 times a week. Excess exercise and poor diet can initiate bone loss in a twenty year old, but with proper diet and exercise you can maintain healthy bones and a healthy immune system throughout life. Current medical advice is to exercise with moderation, avoid marathon runs and workouts which can be depleting and taxing on the bones and heart.

**Herbs**

Eucommia bark has been used for centuries in Chinese medicine to encourage bone restoration. It nourishes the liver and tonifies kidney yang. Drops are made and sold by Dragon herbs, a company run by Ron Teeguarden.

If you like to make tea the following are great to use, barley grass, alfalfa, nettle, rose hips and red clover, black cohosh. Used after menopause and after labor and delivery to replenish the strength of the bones.

Dong quai is a classic female tonic. It is non estrogenic, but helps to balance hormones. Don't take it during menstruation. It is a good herb to use for easing into menopause.

Wild yam regulates hormones, specifically progesterone.

**Supplements**

The current advice is to combine 1,200 mg calcium carbonate to 600 mg magnesium. Take them throughout the day for better absorption. Vitamin D supplementation is critical to those in the northern latitudes. Check on the amount you need, and check your blood levels periodically.

Quercetin supports a healthy immune response, regulates estrogen balance, is anti-inflammatory, and mediates the body's response to stress. You can find quercetin in chlorella, blue green algae and spirulina.

**Bones and Bone Marrow**

**Bones** are a living tissue, constantly creating new bone cells and carrying away old bones cells. Osteoclasts carry away the old and osteoblasts stimulate the new.

*Think of your bones as a structural reservoir of essential life supporting minerals, like calcium and phosphorus.*

**Bone marrow** is the spongy tissue inside our bones. All bones in newborn babies have active marrow, which means they are producing new marrow cells. By the time a child reaches young adulthood, the marrow inside the bones of the hands, feet, arms, and legs stop producing new marrow cells. In adults, active marrow is found inside the spine, hip and shoulder bones, ribs, breastbone, and skull. The bone marrow found in the spine and hip has the richest source of bone marrow cells.

**What does the marrow do?**

Our bone marrow produces blood cells; red blood cells, platelets, and white blood cells. Inside the marrow, blood cells start off as young, immature cells called stem cells. Once they develop, blood cells do not live for a long time inside our bodies. This is why our marrow continuously produces all three types of blood cells to keep us healthy.

The two systems, Bone Marrow and Bone, relate and respond to each other.

A focus on prevention is the Daoist way of attaining health and longevity. Restore your jing chi if you are already showing symptoms of bone loss, and preserve your jing chi as you get older to prevent health problems.

# Bone Packing and Buddha Palms

Bone Packing is the next step in your practice if you have been doing the Bone Breathing Qigong for several months. Review Bone Breathing from Section 1 before you continue to Bone Packing and Buddha Palms. Now that the bone marrow is open and the chi is moving fluidly you can continue the practice by holding, or packing, the chi into the bones with each breath.

Complete the entire Bone Breathing sequence, breathing into all of the bones, and then continue breathing, but hold the chi inside your bones instead of letting go on the exhale. Picture the chi gathering deeply and staying inside the bone marrow. It is necessary that you have done bone breathing to create an open flow of chi throughout all of your bones. The new space that you create with each practice is now ready to accept chi that will fill and enliven the bone marrow. Do approximately 10 breaths of Bone Packing, holding the chi in all of the bones at once, then rest. As the chi is packed into the bones it fills the bones, and is able to wrap the bones and even radiates out to the level of the skin, creating a protective barrier of wei chi. Buddha Palms

An extension of this practice is Buddha Palms. It is called this because we use the palms of our hands to gather and project chi for healing.

After you have done Bone Breathing, continue on to Buddha Palms. (this will take the place of Bone Packing). I find that it is very good to be in a natural outdoor setting for this practice as you are going to be gathering chi from heaven and earth.

## Buddha Palms

*Part 1: Gathering Chi from Heaven and Earth*

1.  Start in a good standing position: Sinking (bending your knees) as you inhale with your palms facing the sky, and push your weight into the ground as you exhale, your palms pressing toward the earth. Your feet are parallel, hip width apart. Smile to the earth and feel it holding you up unconditionally. Feel as if your head is suspended from a string, the weight of your spine is hanging from your head and your hips hanging from your spine. Feel your joints relax.
2.  Begin Bone Breathing until you have opened the space in all your bones. Breath slowly and deeply, synchronizing your movements with your breath, and guiding the chi into all of the bones.
3.  Become aware of the rhythm of your chi at your navel and match the rhythm at the center of your palms, the bottom of your feet, the top of your head, and your pelvic floor.
4.  Raise your hands over your head; palms facing up. Absorb Cosmic Energy (from the entire universe) through your palms, pack this energy inside your bones as you breathe in and let it flow through the rest of your body as you breathe out.
5.  Lower your hands in front of your forehead palms facing out. Absorb Universal Energy (from our Galaxy and the Milky Way) through your palms, pack inside your bones as you inhale and let it flow through the rest of your body as you exhale.
6.  Bring your arms down palms facing the earth. Absorb Earth Energy through the palms, pack inside your bones as

you inhale and let it flow through the rest of your body as you exhale.

7. Drop your thumbs (palms down), bend your elbows and pull the arms back, aligning the 'Tiger Mouth' or LI-4pt. of each hand (fleshy web on back of hand between thumb and index finger), with each hip. Feel the energy passing between the Tiger Mouth points through the hips. Holding the same position of the arms, turn your fingertips to point at your hips.

8. Holding the same position of the arms, turn palms up, fingers pointing forward, the pinky finger side of the hands ('Chi knife') facing the eye of the hips.

9. Release your elbows; bring your forearms in front of you with palms facing up. Relaxing your shoulders; connect and absorb your personal source of power, whatever you like the most in life, whatever gives you enthusiasm (your favorite, weather, people, trees, rhythm, piece of music, etc . . .). Pack inside your bones as you breathe in and let it flow through the rest of your body as you breathe out.

10. Turn your wrists so your palms are facing down, forearms and hands at the height of the navel, connect with the earth, the present moment and whatever allows you to be right here right now, your entire support system. Feel that support and pack it inside your bones as you inhale and let it flow through the rest of your body as you exhale.

*Part 2: Opening the meridians*

11. Bend your elbows; bring your left index finger under your right elbow (left index finger pointing up towards your Heart meridian in your right elbow); right hand above left elbow (right index also pointing upward).

12. Drop index fingers right index points to your Large Intestine meridian in your left elbow, left index points to the ground.
13. Repeat position #11 and #12 (raise and drop index fingers one more time).
14. Holding the 'Chi Ball': Lower your left hand and turn over your palm, to below the navel palm facing up. Bring your right hand over the left, above your navel palm facing down. Feel the Chi between your hands.
15. Open: Move hands away from the lower tan tien, straighten arms, palms down
16. Reverse: Right index finger under left elbow: Repeat positions 11 to 14 with left arm on top of right.

*Part 3: Sending energy to points along the front of the body*

17. With palms down, cross right wrist over left wrist. Energizing the 'Inner Gates' and 'Outer Gates'.
18. Turn both palms up, keeping the wrists together. Energizing the 'Inner Gates' and 'Outer Gates'.
19. Drop the left hand (palm facing up) to below the navel. Turn right hand (palm facing down) above the navel. Hold the 'Chi Ball' right over left.
20. Maintaining contact between the hands (feeling the heat), with left hand remaining below the navel drop thumb of the right hand (opening the 'Tiger mouth'). Slowly move the right hand up the front of the body, (left hand stays below the navel) stopping at all energy centers: Solar plexus, Heart, Throat, and Mid-eyebrow, to open and energize them.
21. Lower the right hand slowly down the front of the body to the navel.

22. Hold the 'Chi Ball'.

23. Bring both palms facing the navel, right over left. Align the center of the palms to send a 'Double beam' of energy to your navel. Feel the warmth spreading in your lower tantien. With your right palm remaining move your left palm up to your solar plexus and energize. Bring your right palm over your left ('Double beam'). Next (right hand remaining) bring your left palm to your heart center, then bring right palm behind left. Continue up to each center, Throat, Mid-eyebrow and the Crown (top of the head). Then go back down the same way you came, left palm first, then the right covering the left for each center.

24. This completes the Buddha Palms practice.

Buddha Palms is a gentle energetic way to strengthen the Conception Vessel along the front of the body. This will encourage the flow of chi up the front of the body for the Women's Water cycle in Microcosmic Orbit meditation.

# Conscious Breathing

## Meditations to clear dampness and disease

### 108 Breaths meditation

This meditation was taught to me by Master Yun Xiang Tseng, known as Wu Dang Chen, a Daoist Priest and internal martial arts master. At a young age, he was chosen to study on Wu Dang Mountain (made famous by the movie "Crouching Tiger, Hidden Dragon") with Master Li Cheng Yu ( a Female Daoist practitioner ) who studied Taoist practices from the age of 10 and lived to be 130 years old. After intensive study, Master Li sent Chen to the United States to share this ancient wisdom and deep knowledge of growing one's personal constitution for success, health and longevity.

The 108 breaths meditation practice moves stagnant damp chi from the lower tan tien, out of the body, creating a healthy alive lower tan tien. As it was taught to me, it transforms Jing to Qi and regulates the mind.

Women will sit with the right leg crossed outside of the left and both hands folded over the lower tan tien; the cauldron which is below the navel. The left hand is placed outside of the right hand with the left thumb pressed into the lau gong of the right hand.

Your breathing will be deep, slow, gentle and even. On the inhale press your tongue to the roof of your mouth and guide the chi from the lower tan tien up the back Du (Governing) channel and down the front Ren (Conception) channel to the lower tan tien. This is one complete circuit of the Microcosmic Orbit on the inhale. Spin or spiral the chi in the lower tan tien, gathering up any stagnation before you exhale.

As you exhale, release the tongue from the roof of the mouth and relax the jaw as you guide the chi up the from Ren channel and out of your mouth. Pull up the perineum to make a complete exhale.

Repeat this breathing pattern 3 times, then take one resting breath (this resting breath is called gentle fire) Repeat the 3 times breathing pattern another 36 times, with one resting breath between. The 3 focused breath cycles with the tongue at the roof of the mouth counts as 3 breaths. The resting breath is not counted. 36 repetitions will add up to 108 breaths and will release post heaven chi from the body. This restores pre heaven chi and is an immortality practice.

You may count any way that is easy for you, by 3 or by 36 sets, or if you are doing this in a group have one person be the counter. It will take about 30 minutes to complete 108 breaths.

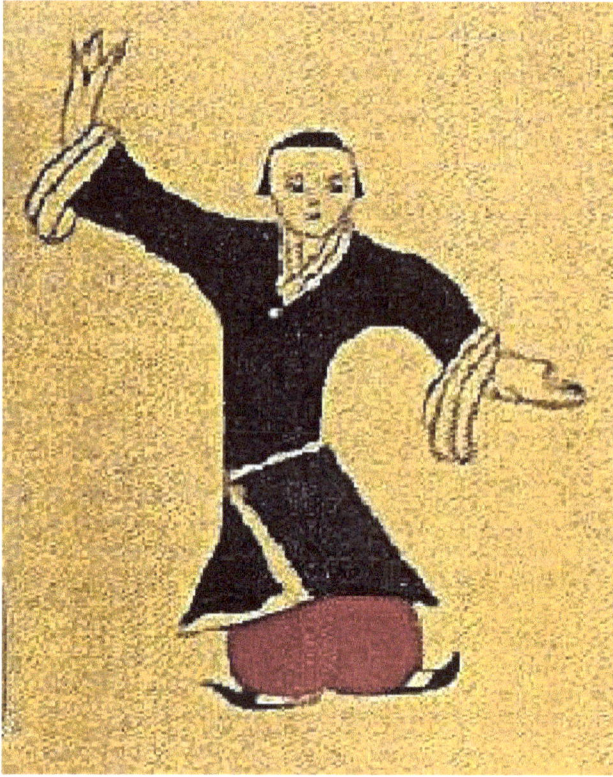

# Tai Chi

Compared to Qigong and Wu Dancing, Tai Chi is a relatively new kid on the block in Chinese history. Many people believe that Taiji Quan was created by Zhang Sanfeng, however, the popular symbol of Tai Chi (Taiji) and the inner martial art of Taiji Quan came from the teachings of his grandmaster, Xiyi Xiansheng Chen Tuan. Chen Tuan lived from 618-907 C.E. He passed on his knowledge of Tai Chi to Zhao Kuangyin first emperor of the Song Dynasty, who trained his soldiers. Zhang Sanfeng lived during the 1200's and visited many Daoist temples and monasteries where he studied. Little is actually known about when or where he died. The Martial Art of Tai Chi is deeply rooted at the Shaolin Temple and Wudang Mountain monastery. Hua Shan mountain, the last place that Chen Tuan lived, is also famous for the Neidan practices. During the 1700s the Chen family became known for their writings and teachings of Tai Chi which blended Martial arts with Daoist breathing and Tao Yin, which came from Chen Tuan. Today there are many styles of Tai Chi, such as Yang style and Wu style.

As a longevity practice for Women Tai Chi is superb in its ability to calm and focus the mind and emotions, and in strengthening the bones and muscles improving the breath. Tai Chi will improve the overall balance of jing, chi and shen. There have been many studies done on the benefits of Tai Chi, including the prevention of Osteoporosis. You can say that Tai Chi is a therapeutic exercise; a defense against disease. It is also more. When you strengthen your framework you provide a container for inner alchemy practices. The Yang supports the Yin.

I first studied Tai Chi in the 1980's with a Chinese American man who had studied at Shaolin monastery. His approach was very strong and he explained each move for its' martial application. I really enjoyed the power and strength that I felt in my body while practicing this form. Fifteen years later I studied with a woman who was trained by Cheng Man-ch'ing in New York City. Her style was much softer, like a dancer, and she exuded joy while practicing. I recommend that if you are interested in learning Tai Chi that you find a good teacher, one who has been practicing for several years.

When I visited China in 2011 I saw a group of women practicing Tai Chi Fan in front of a Confucian temple. This is also a form that I learned and enjoy playing with at times as it resembles Tai Chi and can be done with a group.

Tai Chi aligns with the Taoist philosophy of living in harmony with nature. When one practices Tai Chi gravity is used with proper body alignment to support our physical structure. Like the trigram, humans stand between heaven and earth. Misalignment of our posture affects our organs and consequently our emotions and behaviors. In Tai Chi the eight trigrams represent the Eight Directions.

Tai Chi is first mentioned in the I Ching, Book of Change. In I, there is Tai Chi. Tai Chi generates two extremities. Two extremities generate four aspects. Four aspects generate eight trigrams. One yin and one yang constitute the tao.

*When the body is upright*
*The breath will be smooth.*
*When the breath is smooth,*
*The mind will be still.*

The practice of Tai Chi will bring purification of body, mind and spirit.

An excellent Long Life practice.

# Microcosmic Orbit Meditation

The rendering of the Microcosmic Orbit below was found carved into the wall of a cave around 7th century AD. Word spread among a few hermits on the mountain and eventually the carving was taken to the White Cloud Temple in Bejing.

The Microcosmic Orbit is formed at the first cell division after conception and creates an interface between the physical (post heaven) and spiritual (pre heaven) worlds. It is via this specific Daoist meditation that we can re-familiarize with our primordial (pre heaven) chi.

The diagram of our inner world, which resides at White Cloud Temple, is deep and mysterious, like the mysteries of the universe, and serves as a map for the movement and refinement of chi in our inner world. Our physical anatomy is an inner landscape with its own rivers, forest, mountains, and lakes. Imagine the spine rising to the spiritual peaks of the head and brain.

We begin the journey through our inner terrain at the base of the spine by pumping the water up toward the brain. You see two children pumping a water wheel up toward the kidneys. The cauldron in the lower tan tien symbolizes the alchemical process of refining chi; fire and water practice. Sexual energy that is dissipated can deplete the kidneys. To keep chi from escaping we close the earthly gate (tighten the perineum) and direct the chi upward along the spine to the brain and the upper tan tien where shen (spirit), is refined for leaping off of spiritual peaks to return to the void. There are many messages and lessons along the way, such as the need to cultivate the inner self before the seed of the immortal fetus can be planted; this is represented by the buffalo and farmer.

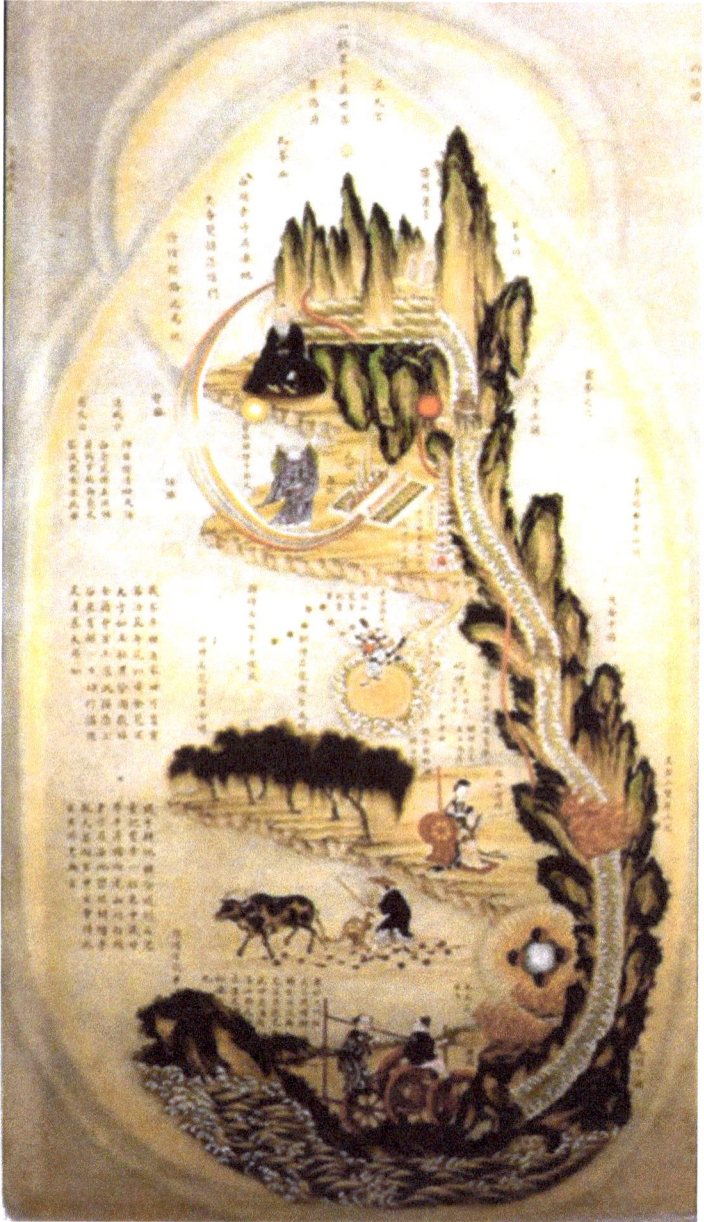

The front and back channels of the microcosmic orbit (the Governing and Conception channels) are prime examples of Yin and Yang energies. When one fuses Yin and Yang, Water and Fire, there is an alchemical response in the body. Moving chi up the front (conception channel) is called the Water cycle; a Yin experience of chi. Guiding chi up the back (governing channel) is called the Fire cycle, accentuating Yang chi.

The lower sea of chi, or elixir field, is an open space which in time will give rise to the lower tan tien. With patient practice, beginning with the breath, the lower sea of chi will create a condensation of chi. This will look like a polished pearl, and this is what is circulated in the microcosmic orbit. It may take a while to create this ball of chi, but it is work the time you invest in sitting meditation practice to experience the opening of these channels. You cannot force it, and when it happens spontaneously there is a sense of deep tranquility.

When I teach a qigong and meditation class I use qigong warmups and seasonal forms to prepare the body/mind for sitting meditation. Before I introduce a meditation practice to a class I attempt to do a little movement or Tao yin stretching prior to the sitting meditation. In this way the mind and body are relaxed and become a conduit for receiving the refined frequencies needed for healing and spiritual development. Meditation relies on the same criteria as qigong: breathing, posture, (upright spine) and awareness.

Meditation is not a competition with the self, it is a spiritual commitment, a point of view in life that becomes important to oneself. If you need 5 minutes a day, or 2 days of meditation, then that is what you should do. I highly recommend that you experience a meditation retreat someday. 2, 3 or 4 days of meditation will accelerate your foundation of experiences and create lasting changes in your awareness. One year I spent a month in a silent meditation retreat in the mountains of Northern New Mexico. There was no cell phone service, wifi, TV, no electricity. We showered outside and slept outside. I was profoundly altered after that month; the worries of the world had no affect on me.

Find a routine that works for you and be consistent. Meditate every day at the same time, if only for 5 minutes. Repetition is the key to success with everything that we do in life.

Sitting meditation relies on breath, posture and focused attention. Let your inhale and exhale be the same length, a circular movement felt by the expansion and contraction of the abdomen. Sit so that your spine is straight, and focus your inner eye on the cauldron in your belly that is smelting the elixir into a pearl of chi.

The inner smile and 6 healing sounds are classic Daoist meditations and often done as preparatory practices leading up to the Microcosmic Orbit meditation. It is critical that in chi circulation the **quality of the chi** is purified. Therefore, the inner smile and 6 healings sounds is an excellent preparation to internal alchemy practices, as it purifies the vibration of the internal organs.

As a foundation practice the Microcosmic Orbit meditation guides chi along the meridians of the front and back of the body. When I say guide, I mean that you use your mind to visualize or direct the chi. With practice you will begin to feel sensations of chi moving. Daoist meditation is not entirely a mental process, but evolves into a felt sense of chi moving. What you can sense and feel you can work with for healing. The quality of chi is essential, and therefore, preparation and refinement of chi is necessary.

Now I will tell you about the **Microcosmic Orbit** meditation. It is the foundation of many Daoist meditations and advanced practices. This practice preceded acupuncture and was used as a way to direct chi in the body to create flow, and health. Acupuncture, which came later, was seen as inferior to positive lifestyle choices and meditation. When chi is flowing in a warm current through the Microcosmic Orbit it will feed the 12 other meridians of the body and support the organs. When the meridians (energetic anatomy) are clear, the deep life force is in flow, unblocked, and able to nurture the body. Universal chi feeds every cell and every space that we know as a living physical body.

Practicing the Microcosmic Orbit meditation on a regular basis will assist you to balance and harmonize the deep river of chi which flows along the front and back of your body. This pathway connects the energetic and spiritual centers of the 3 Tan Tiens, (jing, chi and shen) enlivening primordial chi and refining spirit. The microcosmic orbit meditation will strengthen your spiritual, intuitive and psychic perceptions. Practicing daily will calm the mind, relieve stress and provide you with a deep peaceful sleep. It also develops Wei Chi, protective chi, around your body and the shen is attracted to the jing and chi.

It is recommended that you do 10-15 minutes of physical warm-up before sitting to do any meditation. Qigong is an excellent way to prepare, however, a brisk walk, stretching, Tao Yin, or simply "shaking qigong" is also good. This warm-up allows the blood to oxygenate, the joints to soften and the mind to relax.

**Practice:**
Find a comfortable sitting position with your spine upright and relaxed. Fold your hands over your lower abdomen or place them gently on your knees. Women will place their left hand below the right, thumbs touching, or left hand covering the right if placed over the belly. Take a few a slow deep breaths, allowing your belly to expand on the inhale and contract on the exhale. See a white ball of light forming in your belly, growing brighter with every inhale.

Connect your tongue to the roof of your mouth behind the teeth on hard palate. This connects the Du and Ren channels, or the Governing and Conception vessels. On the next exhale gently pull up the perineum, this closes the earthly gate and creates a complete circuit of the front and back channels. Let your belly relax and expand with every inhale, and pull up the pelvic floor with every exhale.

Focus your mind's eye on the white ball of chi forming in the lower tan tien.

Gently guide this ball of white light on your next exhale, while you gently squeeze the earthly gate closed, up the front channel of the Microcosmic Orbit (water cycle) toward the navel if you are a woman. Continue moving the ball of white light (a radiant condensed pearl of chi) up the front channel to the top of your head and down the back channel, returning to the perineum. See the light in your mind's eye, and feel it as a warm river of chi beginning to move up the front of your body and down the back along the spine.

With each exhale move the ball of chi further up the front of the body until you reach the top of your head, and then begin to move the chi gradually down toward the perineum. After you have made one entire loop, continue to guide the chi along the pathway of the Microcosmic Orbit. Repeat the cycle nine times, and then relax in stillness.

If there is some place along the path that is difficult to see or feel, take a few moments to rest here, relax more. Do not force the chi to move. Adjust your posture if you need to. Let go of any effort or tension. Eventually the chi will move on it's own as the point relaxes and fills with chi. You may feel movement in your body as the chi adjusts.

Continue to focus on your breath and enjoy the feeling of chi moving around your body. Eventually you will drop beneath the use of your mind as the chi circulates. You will be sitting in oblivion, without any effort or need to visualize. Set a timer if you like, or continue in your meditation until your awareness brings you back to your surroundings.

To finish your practice bring the pearl of chi to the top of your head and spiral it clockwise around your head like a galaxy, to clear your mind.

Now guide the pearl to descend and spiral clockwise around the chest, opening and clearing the heart.

Finally bring the pearl back to rest in your belly, spiraling it clockwise and storing it deep inside the cauldron in your lower tan tien. You may use your hands to make a spiraling motion over your belly.

Take a deep breath, stretch and rub your hands together until they get warm. Place your hands gently over your eyes.

Rub your hands together again and massage your face, head, ears, belly, arms and legs. Also massage the meridians of the arms and legs if you have been sitting for a length of time.

**Note:** Always return the condensed pearl of chi to your belly, the lower tan tien. This is highly refined, warm chi and you do not want to leave it in the head or the chest. This is why sitting is the best posture to begin with.

# Ovarian Breathing

In **Ovarian Breathing** you will use your mind's eye to draw the warm vitality of the ovaries into the Microcosmic Orbit. Sexual energy is warmer, more effervescent and lively than the chi we typically circulate in meditation, so it means that special care should be taken to guide this chi properly. Sexual energy is considered Yin in its resting phase, and very creative. Aroused sexual energy is healing and it is important that this chi is circulated and not expended unnecessarily. Therefore, we cultivate a high quality of our chi with the Six Healing Sounds, especially the sound and visualization of color for the endocrine glands, prior to doing Ovarian Breathing.

Ovarian Breathing transports creative and healing energy throughout the body, and especially revitalizes the brain. This practice will also tone the pelvic floor. It is not recommended to do this practice during Menstruation, as the uterus is releasing chi during these days and the ovaries are restoring their chi for the next cycle.

**The Practice:**
Find a comfortable sitting position with your spine upright and relaxed. Fold your hands over your lower abdomen; the lower tan tien. Women will place their left hand below the right, thumbs touching. Take a few a slow deep breaths, allowing your belly to expand on the inhale and contract on the exhale.

Connect your tongue to the roof of your mouth behind the teeth on hard palate. This connects the Du and Ren channels, or the Governing and Conception vessels. On the next exhale gently pull up the perineum, this closes the earthly gate and creates a complete circuit of the front and back channels. Let your belly relax and expand with every inhale, and pull up the pelvic floor with every exhale.

The Ovarian breathing exercise begins with the gentle contraction of the perineum, so gentle that it is like the closing of a flower petal. Bring your attention to the pelvic floor and with a few breaths, begin to feel the opening and closing of the perineum and vagina, relaxing on the inhale and pulling up on the exhale.

Now bring your awareness to both ovaries. (If you do not have ovaries, or a uterus at this time in your life, you did when you were born, and there is still an energetic template of these in your energy field). On each exhale draw the ovaries energy toward the uterus; Ovarian Palace. Fill the Ovarian Palace with chi, see it as a golden white ball, or a pearl of condensed chi. When this pearl is smooth and perfectly formed move it out into the Microcosmic Orbit and up the front of the body, as we did with the Microcosmic Orbit meditation. Guide this chi in a complete orbit up the front and down the back, returning to the Ovarian Palace.

Continue to circulate this ovarian chi, relaxing on the inhale and pulling up on the exhale. It is very important that you return this pearl of chi to the lower tan tien as you complete this practice, and not let it stick in your head or heart. This is why we sit up for this practice, rather than lying down.

With each exhale move the ball of chi further up the front of the body until you reach the top of your head, and then begin to move the chi gradually down toward the perineum. After you have made one entire loop, continue to guide the chi along the pathway of the Microcosmic Orbit.

If there is some place along the path that is difficult to see or feel, take a few moments to rest here, relax more. Do not force the chi to move. Adjust your posture if you need to. Let go of any effort or tension. Eventually the chi will move on it's own as the point relaxes and fills with chi.

Continue to focus on your breath and enjoy the feeling of chi moving around your body. Eventually you will drop beneath the use of your mind as the chi circulates. You will be sitting in oblivion, without any effort or need to visualize. Set a timer if you like, or continue in your meditation until your awareness brings you back to your surroundings.

To finish your practice bring the chi ball to the top of your head and spiral it clockwise around your head like a galaxy, to clear your mind.

Now guide the chi to descend and spiral around the chest clockwise, opening and clearing the heart.

Finally bring the chi back to rest in your belly, spiraling clockwise and storing the white pearl of chi deep inside of you in your lower tan tien. You may use your hands to make a spiraling motion over your belly.

Take a deep breath, stretch and rub your hands together until they get warm. Place your hands gently over your eyes.

Rub your hands together again and massage your face, head, ears, belly, arms and legs.

**Note:** Always return the chi to your belly, the lower tan tien. This is highly refined, warm chi and you do not want to leave it in the head or the chest. This is why sitting is the best posture to begin with.

# Chi Nei Tsang

## Advanced Self Care Routine
*45 minutes, 2 or 3 times a week*

Requires knowledge of the five Elements and the six Healing Sounds.

1. Lie down on your back in a comfortable, quiet place. Bend your knees so that your back is relaxed and your feet are flat on the floor. Put a few pillows under your knees to support them in this relaxed position.

2. Place your hands on your belly and breathe deeply, filing your abdomen first and then let the breath rise up into your lungs. Exhale completely and wait until the next breath comes naturally. Notice any places that hesitate to take in breath and chi. Allow your diaphragm to open in all directions. Feel your ribs soften into the floor and toward the ceiling. If there is tension in taking a full breath, then massage by using your fingers to soften the border of the rib cage so that it may expand further.

Observe any emotion that arises with the breath. Continue breathing with conscious awareness for several minutes. Use the 6 healings sounds to clear emotions that arise from the breathing, or from specific organs. If you are aware of an emotion, rest your hands over the organ that is releasing this emotion and do the 6 healing sounds, and send color into the organs for healing.

3. Use your fingers to feel the texture of the skin inside the rim of your navel. Massage firmly in all directions inside the navel to about 1/2 of the depth of your navel. Allow time for the navel to shift and change; it is connected to all parts of your body via the connective tissue. Feel the energetic connections from your navel to other places in your body. You may use various methods of massage, (circles, pulsing, or simply holding a stretch). Take as much time as you need, this may become a large segment of the self care massage.

4. Move your hands to the lower left quadrant of the abdomen and find the sigmoid and descending colon. Gently pump the large intestine with your fingers. This creates circulation, hydration, intestinal transit and affects the movement of lymph of the pelvis. See the color white filling the large intestine, and use the sound Ssssss to clear away any negative emotions.

5. Continue this technique along the entire length of the descending colon, transverse colon and ascending colon, ending at the cecum in the lower right quadrant of the abdomen. At the flexures of the intestine, under the rib cage on right and left sides, stretch the tissues down to create more space for the breath to move the diaphragm. If there is pain anywhere, pause and breathe, allowing the tissues to respond.

6. Create small circles on your belly with your fingers above the small intestine, moving in larger spirals out from the navel until you have felt the entire area of the small intestine. Feel the natural warmth of the small intestine; this is the fire element and is responsible for extracting the nutrients from our food. See the small intestine filling with the color Red.

Move your hands over your heart and make the sound Haaaaa to release any emotion that puts you out of balance.

7. Explore areas of your belly that call out to you for attention and relaxation; (if you have consistent complaints from your stomach, small intestine, liver and gallbladder, or anywhere else, then spend some time with your hands to massage gently and send healing chi and a smile into the area. Gently lay your hands over all of the organs in your body and fill them with the appropriate colors, and release any unwanted emotions with the sounds. Remember to fill your kidneys.

8. The Uterus lift is beneficial to many women who experience menstrual cramps, incontinence, infertility and painful intercourse. Place both hands with your fingertips near the pubic bone at a 90 degree angle. Sink your fingers down into the belly and then pull the uterus up toward your navel, without sliding on the skin. Your fingers must be anchored into the tissues. You may feel a tugging from the uterus through the vagina, and even a correction in the position of the uterus. Repeat 3 times and then rest your hands, and breathe.

Fill the ovaries and all of your endocrine glands with a purple light.

Chi Nei Tsang can be done anytime during a woman's cycle. However, if you have endometriosis do not do abdominal massage during menstruation as it may irritate endometrial tissue.

8. Rest and return to your breath. Notice the changes that have occurred in your belly and your awareness. Smile.

# Acupressure for Better Sleep and Improved Digestion

I have chosen these two treatment protocol because I see that many women are challenged in these areas. Sleep is so important to overall health and contributes to feeling present and vital. Digestive Fire is essential to long life.

You may wish to review the chapter about Acupressure in Section One of this manual before you begin.

**Recommendations for a good sleep**
- In the evening before bed, Tao Yin meridian stretches
- Belly breath for 5-10 minutes
- Practice the Six Healing Sounds (especially clear the Heart)
- Take a foot bath and massage your feet (get the chi to your heels)
- Eat a light dinner
- Get into bed by 11pm (Melatonin production begins around 9pm)
- Darken your sleeping area and turn off all Wi-fi and phones

**8 Points to use for Better Sleep**
Work on both arms and both legs. The points at the back of the skull are bi lateral; there are mirroring points on each side of the body.
- *Wrist points.* Pericardium 6 "Inner Gate" & Heart 7; "Spirit Gate"

- *On the Sternum.* Conception Vessel 17 "Milk Flow or Sea of Tranquility"
- *Forehead.* Governing Vessel 24.5 "Third Eye Point"
- *Base of Skull.* Bladder 10 "Heavenly Pillar" & Gallbladder 20 "Gates of Consciousness"
- *Heels.* Kidney 6 "Joyful Sleep" & Bladder 62 "Calm Sleep"

## 6 Points for Improving Digestion

Our Fire element (small intestine) is strongest during lunch time Refer to the timetable of meridians. The Stomach, part of our Earth element, is most active at Breakfast. These should be the two biggest meals of our day. Of course, we need to eat clean fresh foods which are full of chi to nourish our bodies. Eat regular meals and relax when you are eating. There are so many food choices at our markets, and many people do not take time to cook, if you are one of these people, then choose fresh unprocessed foods and simplify your diet so that you are not combining too many types of foods at once.

- *On midline of the body on the Belly.* Conception Vessel 6 "Sea of chi" and 12 "Center of Power"
- *On the back, along the spine.* Bladder 21 "Stomach shu" and Bladder 47 "Ethereal Soul Gate"
- *On the outside of the leg, below the knee.* Stomach 36 "Three Mile Point"
- *Bottom of the foot.* Spleen 4 "Grandfather Grandson"

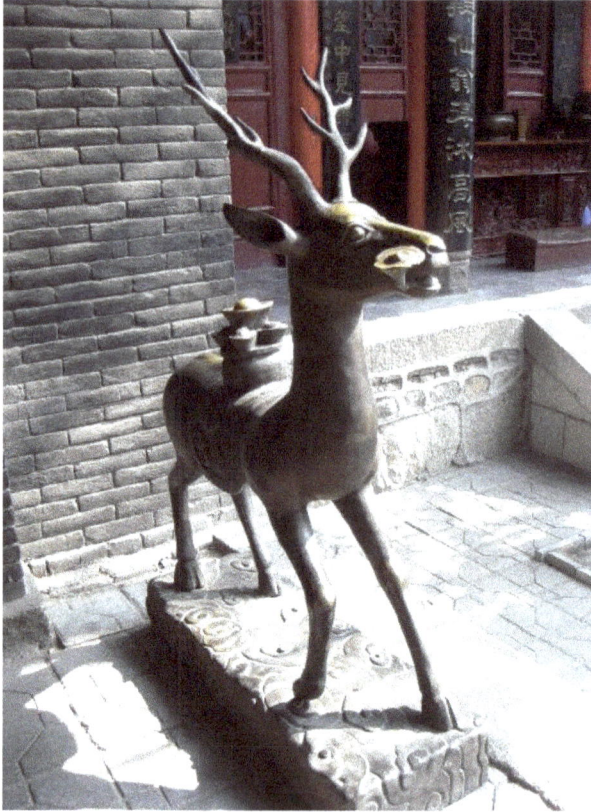

# Daoist Sexual practices

## Inner Beauty, Outer Radiance

*"European alchemy, Japanese geishas, Indian Tantric cults, venetian blinds, fireworks, wedding rings...these and many other disparate technological and cultural features from around the world originated in ancient Chinese sexual practices."*

-Page 1 of Yin-Yang Butterfly, by Valentin Chu.

Sexual energy is a part of all human lives; we are all born from it and have a relationship to it in either a male or female body throughout our lives. Being female brings specific experiences and insights to the ways in which we cultivate and express our Chi. Daoist female sexual practices are specific and beneficial for developing the inner beauty and outer radiance to live a long and healthy life. Whether you are studying *Martial arts* or *Marital arts* there is ample information gathered by the Chinese culture over the past 5000 years to guide you on your way.

All of the Healing and Longevity practices discussed in this book are important in developing an overall healthy body, mind and spirit. The quality and quantity of Chi that is circulating is vitally important to your inner health and your outer countenance. A complete sexual energy cultivation practice will include the Inner Smile and Six Healing Sounds, Breathing and Qigong, Ovarian breathing and Microcosmic Orbit meditation, Breast massage, strengthening the Pelvic Floor exercises and the Orgasmic Upward draw, and a healthy diet. Having a daily practice will smooth out the natural fluctuations of chi that a woman feels during each month. Moderation in all things is a key Daoist practice.

There is no direct translation from Chinese to the word health; the nearest meaning would be to describe a natural, harmonious, balanced individual. Daoist indigenous practices have influenced Chinese Medicine over many centuries. Observations of the lifestyle choices made by a balanced and harmonious human were included in many ancient texts, and included sexual hygiene and behaviors. The Chinese invented paper and the printing press, therefore, more has been written about the movement of the stars and planets and the growth of a fingernail than in any other culture. The abundance of recorded health information developed from the observations of sages and learned physicians from various regions of China was influenced by the philosophy of Daoists. They were keenly interested in sex, health and longevity. Some Daoist practitioners pursued immortality which was underscored by their use of elixirs and alchemical formulas. For most, a long and harmonious life was the goal.

The *"Suwen"* is an oft quoted text and provides some basis for today's Traditional Chinese Medicine practice. Indigenous Daoist practices were adopted by physicians and then became medical theory. *Suwen* describes the balance of Yin and Yang, preventative medicine, sexual behaviors, our relationship with nature, and the importance of longevity. The information recorded in the Suwen probably began as an oral tradition, and was later recorded in conversations with the Yellow Emperor (Huang Ti) and his trusted advisors, about 4th century BC. On sexual matters and immortality his advisors included the Western Royal Mother (His Wang Mu) and her three female attendants; Multi-hued girl, Mysterious girl and Plain girl. Some of these manuscripts were unearthed at the Magwangdui tombs in 1973. The Suwen is considered the root of Chinese Medicine and referred to in Acupuncture training as a valid medical text with important guidelines for lifestyle practices which "Nourish Life" and prevent illness. Chapter 1 discourages sexual encounters when intoxicated. With no direct translation in Chinese for the western word *sex*, we instead see reference to harmonious behaviors between men and women, making sexual intercourse a poetic dance between a man and woman which holds the keys to prolonging life.

Men and women were seen as equal complements to each other, maintaining the Daoist philosophy of the balance of Yin and Yang. Seductive poetry and art abound; a woman's trousseau would include a picture book for the Bedchamber.

The cosmological concept of Yin and Yang, Earth and Heaven, Woman and Man, is embedded in Daoist philosophy, alchemy, science and the Art of the Bedchamber. Balancing these two primal forces of the Universe was the goal to a long life, to live out your **"heaven given"** years. When Yin and Yang are in balance all of nature and humanity enjoy health and peace. Hexagram #63 of the I Ching provides us with the perfect balance of yin and yang; water (female) trigram sits atop fire (male) trigram. The balance of the six yin and yang lines brings us to balance and harmonious completion. This is considered to be the most perfect trigram as all the lines are in their proper location.

**Clouds and Rain**
There are a few fundamental concepts to understand, such as the quality and quantity of chi, the movement of chi through the meridians, and good posture that comes from qigong and tai chi. Once a woman has harmonized her emotions and gathered sufficient chi to circulate, this chi will be guided through the microcosmic orbit. Women need to cultivate their sexual energy whether or not they have a partner as this is all you ever have to bring to a couple's practice. The bedchamber arts have been studied and written about in China for thousands of years. Sex was encouraged for long life, whereas, abstinence and sexual excess were discouraged. The ancient Chinese medical texts always lead you toward balance in your practices and steer you away from extremes.

The Orgasmic Upward draw for women is unique to Daoist sexual practices and requires that you have some familiarity with the Microcosmic Orbit mediation. (see previous chapter on Meditation and Microcosmic Orbit) When the Microcosmic orbit is connected (with the tongue touching the roof of the mouth and the closing of the pelvic floor muscles), the Conception and Governing vessels become the primary meridian which we use to circulate chi that is cultivated in meditation, including sexually aroused chi. This becomes the pathway for circulating Orgasmic chi, in contrast to the typical orgasm which disperses chi. It is better in the long run to conserve and circulate chi, than it is to disperse chi. At the moment just before a complete orgasm the woman will contract her pelvic floor and pump the chi up her spine and through the microcosmic orbit. This action will also allow her to continue experiencing orgasm many more times, each time circulating powerful aroused chi. A woman must have knowledge and practice in using the Microcosmic orbit during meditation so that this becomes a natural guiding of chi during sexual arousal.

From a Daoist viewpoint, sexual and ancestral chi is stored in the kidneys. Our western lifestyles deplete our Yin kidney chi in a variety of ways. The focus of our women's practices is to find a balance between Yin and Yang activity; harmonize the two so that your life experience is even.

Here are a few books that go into great detail on herbs and diet, sexual positions, history and philosophy.

*The Tao of Health, Sex & Longevity*, by Daniel Reid
*Healing Love through the Tao*, by Mantak Chia

*Sex in the Yellow Emperor's Basic Questions*, by Jessieca Leo
*The Yin-Yang Butterfly*, by Valentin Chu

Strengthening the Pelvic floor muscles will contribute to your experience of good health throughout your lifetime without the worries of incontinence. Good tone in the pelvic floor and vaginal muscles will also increase your enjoyment of sex.

*If you are experiencing pelvic pain it is important that you begin with pelvic stretches before you begin strengthening exercises. Look back at the chapter on Tao Yin stretches for some ideas of how to do this.*

**Pelvic Strengthening Exercises**

1. Sitting on a Cushion, with our without a Jade Egg, pull up the pelvic floor muscles. Relax on the Inhale and Contract on each exhale. Pull up on the Exhale. Feel the tailbone moving toward the pubic bone. And feel the sits bones coming toward each other.

2.

   a. Lying on your back, with your knees bent and feet flat on the floor. Pull up the Pelvic floor muscles and with your low back pressed into the floor, lift your head. (you can support your head with your hands) Doing the same, lift one knee.

   b. Keeping your head on the floor, Make the sound SSSSSSS as you pull up the pelvic floor muscles. Also, try other sounds, like Shhhhhh.

c. Lying on your back, bring your knees to your chest. Press your hands against your knees as you exhale and pull the pelvic floor up; tucking the pelvis.

3. Bridge. On your back with knees bent and feet on the floor, lift your butt into the air. More advanced is to lift one leg into the air while your are in bridge. Repeat a few times as is comfortable to your back.

4. On hands and knees, lift and hold opposite leg and arm. Hold for 5 seconds. Repeat on each side several times up to 5 minutes.

5. Squats. Imagine that you are going to sit down on a chair. Engage your pelvic floor muscles and squat. Hold for 5 seconds. Repeat for 5 minutes.

6. Slow marching in place with pelvic floor engaged. Move your arms and legs as if you are marching. Lift the legs as high as you can. Continue for several minutes.

7. Lunges. Hold onto the back of a chair, engage the pelvic muscles and step forward with one leg into a lunge. Hold for 5 seconds and then lunge with the other leg forward. Repeat 5 times on each side.

8. Laying on your back, squeeze a ball or a pillow between your knees, for a minute at a time. Continue several times as you get stronger.

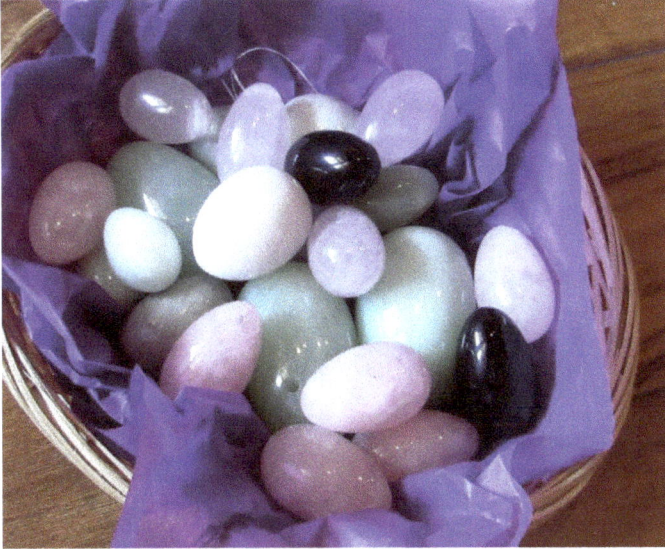

# Jade Egg Exercise

The Jade Egg exercise is both a physical and an emotional experience, which brings benefit to our sexual health as well as to our spiritual understanding of our sexuality. Benefits include better muscle tone in the pelvic floor and more sensation in the vagina. This increases our ability to enjoy sex and also insures the health of our internal organs as they are supported by strong pelvic muscles. Used ritually, the Jade Egg exercise can heal past hurt and trauma.

The Daoists wrote many texts on Sexology; Medical sexology for healing sexual dysfunction, and Inner Alchemy meditations which cultivate sexual essences to accelerate rapid spiritual development, promoting long life. The Jade Egg exercise is an example of Sexual Qigong. Cultivating harmonious emotional chi with the 6 healing sounds, Well breast massage and the Jade Egg exercise are a few of the secrets to long life.

Before using your egg for the first time wash it with soap and hot water. (do not boil it) Rinse the egg before each use. After using your jade egg wash with hot water again, dry and put it in a safe place. A silk bag on your altar is nice.

Preparing to use the egg; cut about one and a half feet of dental floss. Fold it in half and insert the folded end into the egg. Push the string through the egg. When it comes out, open the loop and catch the other end of the string. Tie a knot in the loose end. Use new floss every time.

Lying on your back in a quiet place, begin with breast massage. When you feel lubricated insert the larger end of the egg into the vagina. If you need more lubrication, use some oil you have for the breast massage. Once the egg is comfortably inside of you, use the string to move the egg in and out of the vagina. Use your pelvic floor muscles to pull the egg into yourself on the exhale. The strengthens the pelvic floor muscles. Relax on the inhale, and pull up on the exhale. You can do the Jade egg exercise as often as you like and leave the egg in during the day or night.

Do not use the jade egg if you are menstruating or have any infection. After giving birth wait until all wounds have healed before using the Jade egg. The practice is not recommended during pregnancy, but highly beneficial after birth to tone the pelvic floor.

Regular use of the Jade Egg combined with practices such as Well Breast Massage, the 6 Healing Sounds and Microcosmic Orbit meditation will greatly enhance the quality and quantity of your Chi.

Jade eggs that are used for this practice are drilled end to end to accommodate the dental floss. There are several sources on line. If you are not sure about the source, please contact me. You see in the picture above that several types of stone are used; jade, rose quartz, milky white quartz, obsidian. You will also find calcite and other stones. Pick a stone that resonates with you. Prepare the stone in a special way before using it. If you plan to use the Jade Egg exercise for ritual healing then your will release the egg after using it, such as burying it in the ground.

**Female deer exercise**
This exercise can be done sitting on the floor or on a bed.

Sit so that you can place the heel of hone foot so that it presses into and up against the opening of your vagina. You will want a steady and fairly hard pressure so that the heel presses tightly against the clitoris.

Rub your hands together vigorously. This creates heat in your hands by bring the chi of your body into your palms and fingers.

Place your hands on your breasts so that you feel the heat from your hands enter the skin

Rub with your hands in an outward circular motion, to disperse any stagnation in the breasts.

Continue this circular motion a minimum of 36 times

Tighten the muscle of your vagina and anus as if you were trying to close both openings. Hold these muscles tight for as long as you comfortably can

Relax a moment, then repeat the pelvic floor contractions as many times as feels comfortable.

It is not advised to do this during menstruation or pregnancy.

# Breast Health

Breast Health is total body health. Breast tissues have specific qualities and needs, and have several meridians moving through them. Traditional Chinese medicine views the Conception vessel and Thrusting vessels as having an important influence on the breasts. The conception vessel moves up the front of the body from the perineum and is one of the two vessels joined (with the governing vessel along the back of the body) when one practices the Microcosmic Orbit meditation. The Thrusting vessel originates in the lower tan tien ( in the uterus in women ) and descends to the perineum (huiyin CV-1 ). The two branches of the thrusting vessel ascend upwards from the perineum in the space between the woman's kidneys moving upward in two branches along both sides of the spine into the chest and lungs, ending beside the nostrils. The Thrusting vessels branch out into the breasts as they move through the lungs.

Along with the Conception vessel of the Microcosmic orbit, the thrusting vessels produce the energetic transformations constantly occurring between jing, qi and shen. These are vital pathways for alchemical transformations. The Conception vessel and the thrusting vessels are responsible for regulating the changes in an individual's life cycle. For women those cycles occur every seven years. When these two vessels mature and fill with chi around age 14, the young girl begins menstruation.

"Together, the governing, conception and thrusting vessels are considered to be the energetic gateway of an individual's ancestry, and the link to his or her ancestral skills and knowledge." Jerry Alan Johnson. Chinese Medical Qigong Therapy

Traditional Chinese Medicine looks for the root cause of breast disorders in the spiritual, emotional and mental conditions that support the body's internal organs. Therefore, the 6 healing sounds meditation, qigong and other longevity (yang shen) practices will support overall breast and whole body health. Western medicine also looks closely at a woman's emotional health, diet, exercise, genetics and lifestyle choices in treating and preventing breast disorders. Eat fresh seasonal foods. Avoid sugar, dairy and caffeine which lead to the production of phlegm and can cause breast cysts. This is both prevention and treatment advice.

**Anatomy and Physiology**
The breast is a specialized gland which develops within layers of subcutaneous superficial fascia. The deepest layer forms the posterior boundary and sits over the muscles of the chest wall, the pectoralis major and serratus anterior muscles. Ligaments of Cooper, suspensory ligaments, provide support to breast tissues. The breast contains compartments composed of adipose tissue which vary from woman to woman, and throughout life.

Between the breast tissues and the chest muscles is the retromammary space, which is key to lymph drainage. Wearing a tight sports bra, or other tight fitting bras for many hours a day can limit the movement of lymph in the retromammary space. This creates an unhealthy environment for breast tissues. Lymph drainage is critical to breast health.

Chronic impairment of lymph drainage is implicated in many breast health problems. Lymph flow in breast tissues moves from superficial to deep layers of the breast; into the retromammary space. Supporting breast tissues with a loose fitting bra is important, however, movement is important to the health of breast tissues.

Seventy-five percent of the lymph nodes which drain breast tissue are in the axila (armpit). The other 25% are on the sternum and above the rib cage, or drain toward the rectus abdominis lymphatics.

*Breast tissue* also overlays parts of the latissimus dorsi and the rectus abdominis. There is breast tissue beyond the boundary of the "breast" itself, even into the armpit. Blood flow to the medial and lateral aspects of the breast come via the subclavian artery. Venous drainage originates deep to the areola. Thoracic outlet syndrome can impair circulation to and from the breast and may cause pain and numbness similar to what occurs in the arms and shoulders.

Normal breast changes occur during a woman's lifetime. From the age of 35 onward, the breasts slow the process of replacing lactiferous tissues. The post-menopausal breast is almost entirely fatty tissue. An intermediate stage replaces the lactiferous lobes with dense collagen. Peri-menopausal changes consist of tiny microcysts. While considered normal and not a disease, breast microcysts may be uncomfortable. Between the ages of 40 and 60 there may be benign breast diseases, however at the same time, this is also when malignant breast changes occur.

Having an understanding of one's unique breast tissue is important for each woman. The best way to know what is normal for you is to do regular breast massage. Learn to do a self-massage, or find a massage therapist who has been trained specifically to perform a *Well Breast Massage*. (I created the term "Well Breast Massage" to describe a treatment that is not looking for a problem, but rather supporting healthy touch) I teach this type of massage, and have a companion DVD for those who are interested in learning to care for themselves. The most simple breast massage you can do is to gently circle one breast at a time with your hand in 36 circles, clockwise, then counterclockwise. Then jiggle the breast. Be gentle so that you do not damage the suspensory ligaments.

If you would like to include a Well Breast Massage in your daily or weekly health routine here are some simple instructions: Use a small amount of oil like jojoba (really a liquid wax that does not stain clothing).

**Well Breast Massage Instructions**
*Step 1.* Massage the sternum to stimulate lymph flow.
*Step 2.* Relax the pectoral muscles on the chest and armpit.
*Step 3.* Stimulate lymph nodes in the arms, side of chest, and armpits
*Step 4.* Sweep around the breasts, along the side of the chest, and along the bottom and sides of the ribcage to stimulate circulation in the breast tissue.
*Step 5.* Lift each breast one at a time, then press down gently to encourage lymph drainage into the retromammary space. Then jiggle the breast to increase circulation.
*Step 6.* Swing both arms in a scissoring motion to stimulate lymph flow.

**Medical Qigong** is the oldest of the four branches of Traditional Chinese Medicine and is the source of acupuncture, herbal healing, and massage (tuina). Medical qigong stresses healing from within, and harmonizing our lives with nature. Treatment prescriptions include movement, sounds, meditations and the projection of healing chi into the body. Performing self-care treatments every day for 3 months brings the most effective results in reducing or dispersing breast cysts or tumors. 90 days (3 months) is the time period during which these exercise are designed to transform your internal energy patterns and eliminate the foundation for disease.

**Treatment using Sounds**
1. Sound dissolves the energetic pattern of disease, such as a cyst or tumor. Use a loud sound like "Guo" to purge liver stagnation. Place your hands at the bottom of your rib cage on both sides of the body, (the liver is on the right side). Connect your energy hand into the liver and make the sound Guo while pulling your hands away from the body to release any liver stagnation. Repeat this movement and sound 36 times, several times a day and picture your liver clearing and becoming bright green.

2. Circle both palms around the breasts and picture healing light filling them, then open your arms out to the sides and make the sound "Shang" releasing toxic qi. Repeat this movement and sound 36 times, several times a day.

**Meditation** will reduce stress which weakens the Liver and Kidney Yin which will lead to diseases. The six Healings Sounds is an excellent meditation to practice daily. (find this meditation in a previous chapter). This is a treatment, prevention and a long life practice. Review the Microcosmic Orbit meditation in this book and include the guiding of chi through the Thrusting channels in the same manner as you guide chi in other meridians. I feel the movement in the thrusting channels more as an up and down sensation rather than a circular orbit like the Microcosmic pathway. I have a sense that the Microcosmic orbit and the Thrusting channels create a protective cage around the central channel and the spine.

Overall health depends of good diet, detoxifying sleep and exercise which stimulates breathing. Be sure to sleep 7 or 8 hours every night between the hours of 10pm and 6am to give your body the best chance to detoxify and heal.

**Walking** therapy is also recommended to stimulate the lung channels and clear the emotions, especially around the heart and breast tissues. Qigong practices are also encouraged. I like to do seasonal qigong forms, and forms which focus on specific organs. Movements like walking and qigong are both prevention and treatment. Walk for 15-20 minutes in a quick pace; 60-80 steps per minute. Swing your arms as you walk and visualize healing light filling your chest and breasts. When you are finished walking, stop and feel the chi anchoring in your lower tan tien. Massage your abdomen in slow circles to encourage the chi to descend to your belly. Feel yourself becoming centered and rooted into the earth.

**Acupressure self-care Treatment for Breast Health**
*Point Therapy routine to free Qi flow in the Breasts (find a good point location chart or acupuncture book).* Use this routine as prevention and treatment.

Massage each point for 9-36 breaths.
- *Small Intestine 3 on the side of the hand.* This moves rebellious Qi and Qi depression
- *Stomach 18 underneath the breasts,* Free Qi flow in breasts
- *Stomach 36 on the legs,* regulates Qi in the body
- *Spleen 6 on the inside of the lower leg,* treats breast cysts and tumors. This point is on the liver, spleen and kidney channels.
- *Kidney 1, bubbling spring, on the bottom of the foot.* Hit the center of your foot with your palm and imagine ripples of light and energy flowing up the leg and filling up the lower torso.
- *Gallbladder 21 on the shoulders.* Pat the shoulders. This helps to lower Liver Qi.

**Why Well Breast Massage Is Beneficial To Your Health**
1. Well Breast Massage increases the circulation of fluids like blood and lymph. Since breast tissue does not have muscles to move them, massage is a gentle and effective way to stimulate fluid circulation. Congestion and restriction of movement of breasts from tight clothing is a cause of pain and symptomatic tissue changes.
2. Well Breast Massage eases the discomfort of scar tissue caused from surgery. Lymph flow is compromised around scar tissues.

3. Well Breast Massage supports healthy touch and encourages women to send the message of health and wellness into their bodies as they are performing regular massage. As a result women's attitudes and feelings about their breasts take on a more comfortable status and Well Breast Massage becomes a normal activity

4. The overall tone and fascial structure of breast tissue is supported and strengthened with Well Breast Massage. Breast tissue becomes more alive and vibrant with increased circulation from massage.

5. Women feel empowered with having a technique that is free and effective in eliminating symptoms that are benign. They take responsibility for their health by being informed and educated about their bodies

6. Well Breast Massage is for women of all ages and life experiences. As women age, their bodies and their breast tissues change. Therefore it is important to know what normal change is and how to address symptoms that are outside of normal.

7. Well Breast Massage can become the turning point in a healing regimen as it increases the speed and comfort of healing. The pain and discomfort experienced from various health conditions is eased significantly with healthy touch and movement of tissues.

At some time in our lives we have experienced a degree of breast discomfort, anxiety, trauma or surgery. Massage therapy is an effective "wellness" treatment for breasts because it provides good circulation and tissue mobilization. Touching also helps in alleviating the fear associated with "normal" breast changes. Massage will help to ease many symptoms, prevent more serious problems and will speed healing after surgery.

**Indications for Well Breast Massage**
- Congestion, Edema, Lymph-edema
- Painful Breasts, Pre-Menstrual Tension, Swelling or Tenderness
- Discomfort due to Pregnancy, Breastfeeding, or Weaning
- Drainage Problems due to Large Breasts
- Tenderness due to Benign Conditions or Normal Breast Changes with Aging
- Pain or Trauma after Surgery or Biopsy
- Scarring or Piercing
- Discomforts related to Cancer Treatment*
- Better Self-Image
- To Become Familiar with Normal Breast Changes

**Precautions and Contraindications**
- Mastitis, Post Surgical Infection, or Any Active Infection
- Do Not Massage Implants that are Painful or Distorted in Contour
- Do Not Massage Any Undiagnosed Lump
- Do Not Massage a Tumor or Abscess

*wait a few weeks after chemotherapy or radiation treatment to do Well Breast Massage and do not massage on any undiagnosed lump or on a tumor or abscess

*Prevention is always the best medicine.*

# Tao Yin

Tao Yin (or Dao in) is the Chinese word for physical energy directing. Using one's mind-eye-heart we direct chi for opening the flow through the Meridians, thereby bringing ease of movement to the body, and a balanced interaction between the organs of the physical body.

Thousands of years ago the people living by the Yellow River developed movement practices to enhance a healthy and long life. People lived simply, they sat but had no chairs, they ate but had no tables. Just as we experience today, too much repetition can create stagnation, poor health and pain. For thousands of years people have been guiding chi. Wise people like Chen Tuan developed postures to counter repetition and bring more fluidity into the mind and body. He was also mindful of the movement of the seasons and developed movements that harmonized the human body with the body of nature. Some of these movements appear to mimic the movements of animals, others look like yoga postures. The five animals we see imitated in Tao Yin are the tiger, deer, bear, monkey and the bird. All Tao Yin postures are meant to gently stretch open the meridians while not overstressing any joints or ligaments, as compared to Indian Yoga which focuses on opening the Chakras. Using your breath to complete the extension of chi is key to making these movements successful and enjoyable. Hold a pose for 5 or more breaths, being certain not to create any pain. Allow the breath to move into the meridian and guide the chi to move with your minds eye.

In modern day terms we could say that this type of gentle exercise will reduce stress and energy blockages. Tao Yin is an excellent this to do at the end of a day to bring balance to repetitive postures that you have held. It is also a great warmup in the morning to enliven the body before you start your day. Tao Yin can be done by anyone, at any age, and with all health backgrounds. It is very gentle and can be done sitting or lying on the floor, or sitting in a chair. In China, Tao Yin is prescribed for healing and prevention of disease. Among Daoist practitioners self-massage and Tao Yin are a common practice after long periods of sitting meditation. Enjoy the benefits of Tao Yin if you have been sitting too long at a desk, standing for work, have been ill and lying down a lot, riding in a car, or sitting a long time in meditation.

A record of many Tao Yin moves is found in the Taoist Canon which was compiled in China between 1436 and 1449 A.D. During the Tang Dynasty 652 ad, Tao Yin became an official part of Court Medicine. The famous physician, Sun Simiao (581-682 AD) compiled "Prescriptions of a thousand ounces of gold" in which he outlined many qigong and tao yin prescriptions.

Chen Tuan (born 870 A.D.) was a student of Li He, who was a student of Yin Xi, and Yin Xi was a direct student of LaoTzu. Chen Tuan, known as the dreaming priest, perfected Taoist Dream practice and sometimes slept for hundreds of days at a time. He was also a respected sage who performed divination practices at the court for emperors. His chi had to be clear and supple to achieve all that he did. The gentle stretching postures of Tao Yin allow fluidity to return to the connective tissue which encompasses the meridians.

Lao Tze (500 bc) called it regulating the respiration. Some say the Lao Tzu lived to be 260 years old. Lao Tzu says in chapter 76 of the Tao te Ching,

*When people are alive,*
*Their bodies are soft and supple.*
*When people die,*
*They are stiff and hardened.*
*When tree, grass and animals are alive,*
*They are soft and pliable.*
*When they are dead*
*They become dry and brittle.*

 Tao Yin:
1. Harmonizes and guides the chi through the mind/body
2. Supports the tendons and joints
3. Relaxes the psoas and diaphragm
4. Improves flexibility
5. Releases toxins via the breath
6. Strengthens the lower tan tien

You do not need to know all of the meridians to receive the benefits of Tao Yin. Guide the chi with your intention, and it will move during the resting phases. Chi, or energy, is able to be guided like this. Your active intention and each posture initiates the yang phase and uses the breath to stretch the body. The resting yin phase allows the chi to move where you have guided it. Take a resting breath or two between postures and enjoy the feeling of chi flowing in your body. Your spirit will be more content when your body is relaxed. Breathe deeply by letting the abdomen expand on the inhale and pull up the perineum on the exhale, in this way you strengthen the lower tan tien.

Hua Ching Ni says to imagine you have been lying in a cave for a thousand years, you are completely relaxed and as you wake up you realize that you are a spirit who has awakened in a physical body. You take a deep breath and begin to make physical movements. There is no rush, slowly turn your attention to the life force in your body.

There are many postures and movements that you can choose from, it is not necessary to do them all. The goal is to rebalance your chi and harmonize your mind and body. Imitate the flow of water, or bamboo moving in the wind. Sit like a tiger resting in the grass, and stretch like a dragon reaching for heaven. I have written the following for you as an easy introduction to some of the Tao Yin postures.

*Begin with Conscious Breathing.* Lying on your back, smile and breathe in golden light to your face, heart and lower tan tien. Place your hands gently on your belly and feel the expansion of your breath. Then place your hands on your chest and feel the movement of breath here. As you move into each posture, stay there for three to five breaths.

1. *Pericardium and Kidney meridians*
Laying on your back. Flex the soles of your feet and make a fist as you inhale. Press your fingers into the Lao Gong point in the middle of your palm as you make the fist. Guide the chi up from the bottom of your feet to flow around the heart. As you exhale relax your fists and relax the feet. The chi flows back down and out the soles of the feet. Sometimes this is called the

Lotus Fire and Water meditation. Imagine the sun above your head filling your heart, and the water below you coming into the soles of your feet to fill the kidneys. Your heart is the lotus flower and your kidneys are the lotus bulbs.

### 2. Kidney and Bladder Meridians

Stretch out like a starfish with your hands above your head and your legs open like a V. Stretch one arm, then one leg, the other arm, then the other leg so that you open the space around the kidneys. As you reach out in all four directions you open the space around your kidneys for chi to flow in. This is a wonderful stretch for anyone who is yin deficient or having hot flashes.

Bring knees up toward your chest and reach thru the knees to grab the ankles. Let the legs fall open to stretch the kidney meridian.

Hug your knees into your chest and gently rock from side to side.

Sit up with legs straight, and spine lifted up. Move your chin toward your toes to stretch the bladder meridian.

### 3. Liver and Gallbladder

Sit with both legs extended to the front, opened into a V as widely as is comfortable. Do not raise the knees, but keep them attached to the floor. Keeping the spine erect (not rounded) reach forward until you feel a stretch in the liver meridian.

Lying on your back again, bring the knees up to the chest, hug them in and then let them fall to one side, stretching the GB meridian. Arms rest flat on the floor and the head looks away from the bent legs. Then let them fall to the other side as the head looks the opposite direction.

*4. Lung and Large Intestine*
Standing or kneeling or sitting, clasp hands together behind the back and lean back, looking up. Then come forward bending to the floor with the arms and shoulders opening forward, hands are still clasped. Change thumb position and try it again. 3 deep breaths

Cross your legs in a seated position and reach both hands over your head. Turn your palms to face the sky. Look up.

*5. Spleen, Stomach and Pancreas*
Fold one leg in front of you and stretch one leg out behind you like a tail. Keep the spine moving forward. (pidgeon pose). Change to the other leg. Take 3 deep breaths.

*6. Heart and Small Intestine*
Sit with legs open wide, the knees bent and the soles of the feet together. Hold the hands around the toes, and bring the feet in toward the body as much as possible. Then, slowly bend forward trying to touch the forehead toward the thumbs.

With the same leg position, lean forward and look to one side, twisting the spine. Then look to the other side.

*7. Hip Opener. Preparation for sitting meditation*
Cross your legs and arms and bend your head toward the floor. Breathe, and change the leg and arms positions, to fold over

again. As you come up into a seated position you will feel your sits bones balanced on the floor.

Gently shift your awareness inside to your breath for meditation.

# Eating for a Long and Healthy Life

What you choose to eat is very important for good health. Daoists honor the physical body as much as they do the spiritual body. The human body is a microcosm of the macrocosmic universe; everything found in nature can be found inside of our physical bodies. Jing, Chi and Shen (essence, energy and spirit) are the three treasures which define our physical existence and must be kept in balance and harmony to achieve a long and healthy life. Postnatal Jing (the raw physical essence that we maintain after birth), must be nourished specifically with the right foods and herbs to maintain vibrant chi. This gives rise to the chi and shen which can find a temple within the body to call home. "The body is the temple of life. Energy is the force of life. Spirit is the governor of life. If one goes off balance, all three are damaged." Wen-tzu classic (first century BC)

As we age our digestive fire can become weak and therefore we must choose foods and herbal supplements that boost our digestion and provide our bodies with the chi that is necessary for an active life. Think of food as preventative medicine. Your food choices will either nourish jing and improve your level of chi or decrease it. The more high quality chi you have, the more vitality there will be in your organs. Our organs manifest emotions which guide our behaviors. When our physical body is nourished and in balance we are naturally able to balance our emotions and our decisions in life. Traditional Chinese Medicine advocates a diet that is based on fresh, organic, seasonal foods.

### Five Elements Eating

*"In the long history of Chinese medicine, we have observed that each person is born with an elemental constitutional type that manifests certain physical and emotional attributes. Eating foods that benefit and correspond to your particular type in the Five Elements archetype helps to maximize health and balance your body, mind and spirit."* Page 41. *Second Spring* by Dr. Maoshing Ni

The five elemental constitutions are the same five elements that we find in the cycles of Nature; Wood, Fire, Earth, Metal and Water. Each type has gifts and vulnerabilities, which means that what is right for you to eat may not be right for someone else. Eating seasonal foods has the greatest influence on your health according to TCM. Seasonal fresh foods will nourish your body and help you to adjust to the change in the seasons, aligning your body with nature. The wisdom of the five elements guides our food choices throughout the seasons.
Each of the five elements is associated with a taste or a flavor that produces a therapeutic action on the organs in our bodies. There is also a natural way to prepare foods that are available during each season. The flavor of Sour in the Spring is said to be absorbed by the liver and gallbladder. Although the foods that are growing fresh in spring have more of a bitter quality to them that aids the liver, the *flavor of sour* would be used to bring the liver back into balance. Foods that grow easily in summer are spicy and hot which causes the body to sweat. If your fire element is out of balance you would choose to add *bitter flavors* to your diet.

The five flavors should be balanced with each meal to stimulate the organs and the flow of chi throughout the body.

Eat fresh foods of the season and use the wisdom of the five flavors to bring balance back into the body if your constitution needs it. You will notice in the graph below that there are preferred ways of preparing foods in each season that matches the needs of the weather and of our bodies. For more information on this topic I recommend that you get a copy of Paul Pitchfords book, "Healing with Whole Foods." This is an excellent resource book which features Oriental traditions and Modern Nutrition, including seasonal recipes and ways to balance your individual constitutional needs.

*Review the information on the five elements in the chapter on the six healing sounds to refresh your memory of the emotions that are expressed in the organs.*

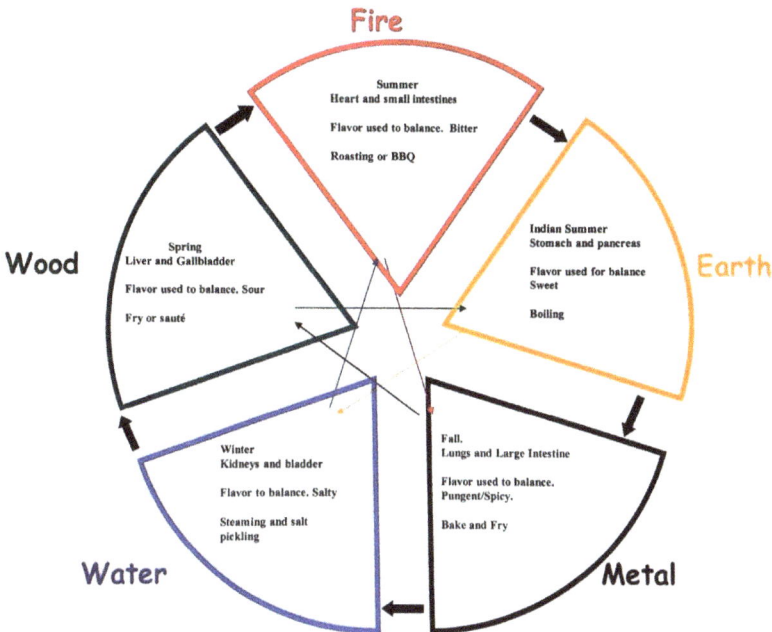

Fire

Summer
Heart and small intestines

Flavor used to balance. Bitter

Roasting or BBQ

Wood

Spring
Liver and Gallbladder

Flavor used to balance. Sour

Fry or sauté

Earth

Indian Summer
Stomach and pancreas

Flavor used for balance
Sweet

Boiling

Winter
Kidneys and bladder

Flavor to balance. Salty

Steaming and salt pickling

Water

Fall.
Lungs and Large Intestine

Flavor used to balance.
Pungent/Spicy.

Bake and Fry

Metal

C 2019 Caryn Diel

# Herbs and Medicinal Mushrooms

Chinese herbal medicine is one of the oldest and best researched areas of wellness in the world. Medicinal mushrooms and herbal remedies work synergistically with each other to bring the best result. Cooking with fresh mushrooms and herbs is a great way to receive the benefit of their medicine. Add them to almost any recipe, cook them into a broth or tea, take as a tincture, or as a supplement in capsule form. Herbs and Fungi (mushrooms) used in the diet will maintain the immune system and provide overall health and longevity. Consult a trusted herbalist or mycologist to choose the correct combination for you.

Two herbs that have a long history of being beneficial for women are Codonopsis (sometimes called the poor man's ginseng), and Dang gui.

"**Codonopsis** is one of the most famous and widely used Chinese tonic herbs. It is very mild and without any side effects, yet it is a superb and potent Qi tonic. It invigorates the Spleen and Lung functions so that Qi is replenished, and it promotes the production of body fluids. Codonopsis is also an excellent blood tonic and a major immune system tonic. Codonopsis is extremely effective at boosting vitality and relieving a sense of general fatigue. Many women use it to build blood.

Codonopsis is rich in polysaccharides that are beneficial to everyone. These immune boosting polysaccharides have been shown to be useful in supporting the immune systems of older people as well. Codonopsis is believed to have an action similar to that of Ginseng, but gentler. It is often used in place of Ginseng in traditional formulas that actually call for Ginseng to be used as a main Qi tonic, especially when the purpose of the formula is to invigorate the Spleen and Lung functions." Ron Teeguarden of Dragon Herbs.

Codonopsis is a great herb to use when there is a lack of appetite. It is also helpful in strengthening organs that have experienced prolapse from childbirth or aging. As a tonic herb it will stimulate the growth of white and red blood cells. It lowers blood pressure, and regulates blood sugar. It has been used to treat fatigue and weakness of the limbs, and shortness of breath or chronic cough.

**Dang Gui** is one of the most commonly used herbs in the Chinese herbal system. It is primarily known as a "women's herb," though many men consume it as well. Most famously and importantly, it known as a superior blood tonic, and that is one reason women use so much of it. It is also used conjunctively as a "blood vitalizer," meaning that it supports healthy blood circulation, especially in the abdomen and pelvic basin. Men and women benefit from superior circulation. Dang Gui is very widely used to help establish, support and maintain healthy menstrual balance in women. It also has analgesic and mild sedative (calming, relaxing) actions." Ron Teeguarden of Dragon Herbs

Food is considered a supreme tonic; herbs can be used with foods you are preparing. For example, you can cook dang gui and use the liquid that is left over to cook your rice into a congee.

"The China Study" by Campbell and Campbell, 2006, is an excellent resource book for learning about current eating trends among the Chinese population. This book gives us a modern look at the diet of most people in China today, and the absence of diseases which manifest from their diet. Women take notice of this, "Findings from rural China showed that reducing dietary fat from 24%to 6% was associated with lower breast cancer risk" page 87 China Study. The average age of menarche in China is seventeen years, as compared to eleven year in the U.S. Clearly, diet matters.

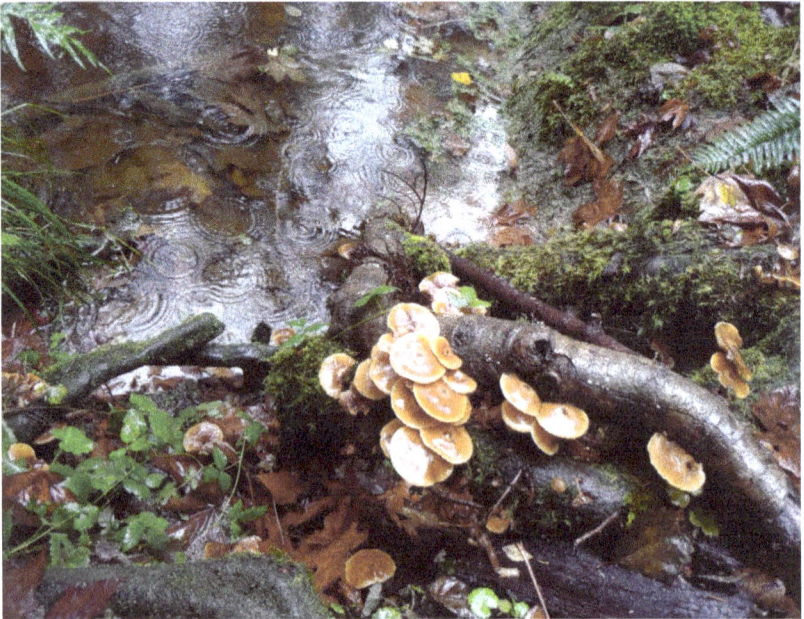

Medicinal Mushrooms (fungi) have been used for centuries in China along with numerous wild harvested and cultivated herbs. Many mushrooms can be added to your diet and are easily available in grocery stores. Mushrooms must be cooked! Cooking breaks down the chitin layer so that the polysaccharides are available to boost our immune function. Oyster mushrooms, Lions Mane, Turkey Tail, and Reishi are perhaps the best known and easiest to find growing wild in the Pacific Northwest. Shitake is also well known and can be cultivated at home.

**Oyster Mushrooms** contain lovastatin and mevinolin that reduce cholesterol levels and pancreatitis inflammation. This mushroom is one of my favorites. I add them to scrambled eggs. Oyster mushrooms relax and improve your mood, (contains B6) improve skin quality and lower your cholesterol. They contain high levels of zinc and iron. Most grocery stores carry fresh and dried Oyster mushrooms.

**Lions Mane** (named for its appearance) is used in TCM for digestion and gastric ulcers, nerve issues and general debility. It contains brain neuron growth factor compounds that cross the blood brain barrier. Lions Mane reduces depression and anxiety, may prevent dementia, reduces tremors and may have positive effects on other neuro muscular conditions. Overall a good mushroom to improve memory, boost concentration and protect your nervous system. Easy to add to your favorite recipes.

*Fun Fact*
The discovery of nerve growth factor proteins is credited to a woman, Italian scientist Rita Levi-Montalcini, and earned her the 1986 Nobel Prize in Physiology and Medicine. She lived for more than one hundred years.

**Turkey tail** has a beautiful fan shape. It has been used for infections and inflammation in the body. It is a good adjunct with chemotherapy and radiation. It is anti-viral, immune modulating, analgesic and anti-inflammatory. Often found in cancer treatment protocols because it has the ability to regenerate white blood cells. Use Turkey Tail to treat the common cold, aid your digestion, and to heal infections. It has a tough texture and needs to be boiled in water for a couple hours to make a broth. Or you can find capsules and tinctures on line.

**Reishi** the Queen of Mushrooms, also known in China as the mushroom of immortality, is found growing in the PNW, however it is time consuming to prepare and is not usually eaten with food. Reishi is well researched and has been used in China for more than 4000 years. It will help you to sleep better, stress less and cures seasonal allergies. You find Reishi in many tinctures in combination with other fungi that assist the body to breathe more easily and relax the heart. It is adaptogenic, helps with circulation, and also assists in hormonal balance. Find a good tincture.

"They dose themselves with the germ of gold and jade and eat the finest fruit of the purple polypore fungus...by eating what is germinal, their bodies are lightened and they are capable of spiritual transcendence." Wang Chung 100 AD.

**Shitake** is well known and easy to find at the grocery store. This mushroom is traditionally used for increased stamina, circulation, arthritis, diabetes, high cholesterol and immune deficiency. This is a delicious medicinal mushroom to add to stir fried vegetables. You will find them in capsules and tincture form also. Studies have shown that it improves immunity, reduces inflammation and has positive effects on the cardiovascular system. Shitake supports your liver, lowers cholesterol and gives you glowing skin. It is called a superfood because it contain seven of the nine essential amino acids.

Chinese dietary and herbal wisdom has a vast history, much of it recorded and disseminated for thousands of years and, more recently, researched. In a nutshell, the Daoist approach to good diet is to eat seasonally and in moderation. Avoid big meals, especially late at night. Keep Jing, Chi and Shen in balance. Realize that your organs manifest emotions that lead to thoughts and behaviors. A balanced constructive life includes food, exercise, sleep and time in nature and with friends and family. If you are seeking better health and vitality with your food choices, do some research and talk to nutritional experts. Get the advice of a TCM doctor about your specific strengths and weaknesses, and set realistic goals. The dazzling array of foods in our markets does not lead us to any sensible conclusion about what to eat or how to prepare foods that best suits our individual needs.

Not all Chinese are Daoists, but the philosophy of Daoism runs deep in the veins of the Chinese people, and there is a saying that all Daoists are physicians. Chinese culture is based upon the structure of Daoist thought. Devoted Daoist practitioners avoid meat, alcohol, tobacco. Some follow a vegetarian diet. They eat simply and listen to their body. Above all use moderation, choose fresh foods and honor the source of those foods.

*What is good for your heart is good for your digestive fire.*

# Second Spring

In Traditional Chinese medicine, the time after a woman ceases the flow of Heavenly Water, (menstruation), is called her Second Spring. The passage into Menopause may take several years and include many physical and emotional changes. With conscious care of your mind and body this transition can be smooth. This is a transition that began when you were born, an example of constant change. According to the Nei Jing, Second Spring is the third important phase in a woman's life. A woman's life is measured in cycles of seven years. Seven times seven is forty nine, a time when the body begins to slow down the aging process by stopping menstruation. This is a time to be diligent with meditation practices which guide chi into the eight extraordinary vessels, such as the microcosmic orbit and thrusting channels. With the cessation of the monthly loss of blood a woman becomes more yang, and this may be a time of great achievement and independence.

Some women feel as sense of new freedom during their second spring. Whatever age you are, it is possible for you to regenerate, renew and revitalize yourself. Your total health depends upon physical vitality, emotional balance, mental creativity and spiritual connection. I have experienced exceptional health and vitality into the later years of my life because I have followed the Daoist practices outlined in this book, been willing to learn new things, and adapt to new situations. Today I feel great, have no pain or disease and sleep 8 or 9 hours every night. Learn to slow and reverse the aging process by practicing some of what is offered in this book every day. From the Chinese perspective a mature woman is a family and community treasure, her experiences and inner resources are to be enjoyed and shared with the world. For most women the Second Spring of life is a time of fewer distractions, deep appreciation of life and new self-understanding.

As you enter menopause your body produces fewer hormones, such as estrogen and progesterone that maintain the health of your bones and the fluidity in your connective tissues. The consequences of having fewer hormones available to your body could be osteoporosis, heart disease, wrinkled skin, lowered vitality, inability to sleep, mood changes and decreased libido. These are not conditions to look forward to, however, they can be approached with grace and support. Consider this time of your life as a normal, healthy transition. The aging process invites us to value our experience, inner growth and wisdom, and to find ways to maximize our health and happiness. Daoist practices offer you many ways to strengthen your physical, mental, emotional and spiritual body. Changing the foods that you eat, your daily routine and your perspective of life may be what is needed, and the good news is that aging has been honored and studied in China for centuries, so there is ample advice available to you. It may be fun to find new things to bring into your life, especially if you look and feel better.

Did you know that in China birthdays are not celebrated until after the sixtieth year of life? Older people are highly esteemed.

Nurture your Three Treasures: Jing, Chi and Shen (essence, energy and spirit). Cultivating the balance of your physical essence, energetic chi and spiritual being has been part of Taoist anti-aging tradition for more the five thousand years. Daoist meditation practices guides you to align with your original chi and brings you into the stillness and silence of the Tao.

If your life is divided into three parts, the first third of your life is a focus on jing, or physicality, growth and reproduction. The middle of life is about chi and expressing your energy. Second spring is a time of the last third of life which begins a focus on shen, your spiritual growth. The balance of jing, chi and shen will affect the chemistry of our bodies, the health of our organs, and the choices that we make.

This is a new season in your life, embrace it completely with an inner smile.

I recommend that you get a copy of Dr. Mao's book, "Second Spring." It is loaded with simple, quick Chinese beauty and food tips to energize your mind and body.

# SECTION 3

# Immortality

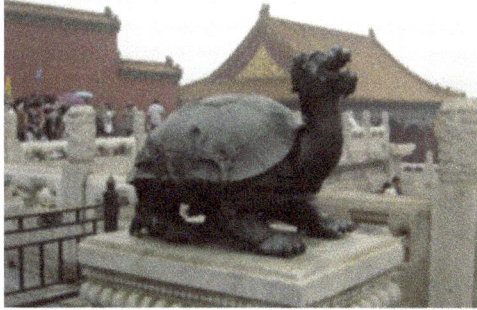

Your immortal soul is much older than your body and mind, it resides in the stillness of creation. The Tao represents infinity which is difficult for our physical mind to understand. However, there is a part of your being and consciousness that resides in the Tao, and as you settle into stillness your begin to experience the yin and yang of motion and stillness. Motion creates all things; it is the life in all things, it is the fragrance and the sensation that moves inside of the body and mind. Your immortality is already guaranteed. You are an immortal being within the Tao.

The Jade Emperors Mind Seal Classic tells us that the secret of immortality is this:

> *Keep to nonbeing, yet hold on to being*
> *And perfection is yours in an instant.*

This instruction is simple but not easy to perfect in a world of physical duality.

**How did ancient Daoists seek immortality?**

Is immortality the state of refined consciousness that reunites with the universal chi field at the moment of our physical death? Or is it the actual length of a life calculated in years? Can nature show us the way of immortality, or is it found in a magical elixir? Ancient Daoists looked for a path, a way, to re unite with the Dao, thus completing the circle of returning.

Attracting immortality is a Daoist concept that became a highly organized system of practices and rituals during the Tang Dynasty (618-907BC). This was the golden age in China for Art, Literature and Daoist practices. During this time in Chinese history adepts had formal guidance in how to consciously integrate healing, longevity, and immortality into a complete system of spiritual attainment. Practices such as stilling the mind and absorbing chi have become part of the Daoist pathway to immortality.

For many Daoist practitioners this was not the goal, they were content with Longevity, however others chose to retreat to mountains and caves in order to refine their minds and bodies to a lighter and freer state of chi. Legends tell us that these spiritual adepts, like Sun Bu'er, hermits, alchemists, and herbal masters like Ho Hsien Ku, would ascend to the clouds as immortals in broad daylight. Indeed, the Chinese image of mountain translates to immortal.

**How can we apply ancient concepts and practices to our lives today?**

We learn from famous Female Daoist immortals like Sun Bu'er that eliminating obstacles and distractions is one of the first steps along a path to immortality. She may not have been able to imagine what numerous distractions we have in our highly compressed busy lives at this time on the planet, but she was well aware of the daily distractions of living which challenge one's ability to conquer a busy mind. Indeed, setting aside a consistent time during a busy daily schedule seems nearly impossible for most people today. It can be accomplished, but requires a deep and sincere intention to be successful. The focus has to be clear and succinct with realistic goals. Progress may be gradual, and so it should be in order to balance and harmonize family and work lives. Time out for focused practice can be found in attending an annual retreat for oneself. Progress during retreats can bring sudden clarity and lasting achievement to our sustained efforts. Even Sun Bu'er delayed her commitment to immortality practice until after she had raised a family and found a suitable teacher. Simplification is the key to living a lifestyle that brings spaciousness into each day and aligns us with the Dao.

Integral to Daoist thinking is an appreciation of the simple and the profound, the large and the small, the complementary movement of yin and yang. In this section there are advanced practices which rely on a foundation of basic practices found in sections one and two. The classics, Tao de Ching and I Ching, are included in the immortality section, and could rightfully be placed in the beginning sections of practices for Women as they constitute the distillation of the best of Daoist philosophy which guides life. Our beliefs often guide our behaviors, and as the yin and yang of it would tell us, sometimes our experiences will mold our beliefs. Therefore, if you decide to study I Ching and Tao de Ching you will find that the poetic and often metaphoric wisdom will assist you to refine your immortal soul, and guide you in how to adapt to change in a quickly changing world. If you have found comfort and vitality from the healing/curing and longevity practices you will in time come to appreciate the profound concepts in these two beloved Chinese classics.

*Live a long and youthful life, and be of benefit to humanity.*

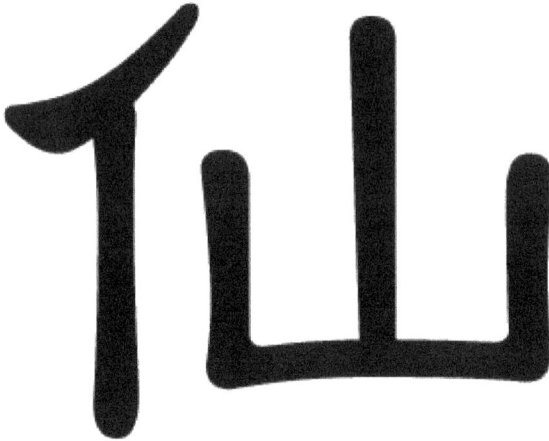

Whatever degree of immortality is being considered, the concept of immortality is integral to all of Daoism. During the Tang dynasty the Masters Sun Simiao and Sima Chengzhen emphasized that the ultimate goal of Daoist practices was the complete transcendence of worldly states with the final goal of immorality. Healing and Longevity exercises played an important part and appear in various levels of the immortality curriculum.

Now that you are familiar with the cultivation of your personal chi, let's connect with the cosmic and universal chi of creation and absorb the chi of nature. This is the next step in refining your body and spirit.

# Immortality concepts from the Tang Dynasty

*"Humans need to be aware that their own existence is an integral part of limitless time and the universe." Zhuangzi*

Sun Simiao and Sima Chengzhen produced many written records on healing exercises which appear in various levels of the immortals curriculum.

> "The first and maybe most important master of longevity in the Tang is Sun Simiao 孫思邈, born in 581 near the western capital of Chang'an. According to official biographies, which tend to stereotype masters as child prodigies and emphasize personal virtues, such as bone-deep honesty and a hesitation to accept imperial honors, he was a precocious child who studied eagerly from an early age. By age twenty he supposedly not only had an extensive knowledge of the classics and philosophers, but was also familiar with Buddhist and Daoist scriptures. Despite several invitations to serve at the imperial court under the Sui and early Tang dynasties, he went to live in seclusion on Mount Taibai 太白山 in the Zhongnan mountains, about a hundred miles from his ancestral home.
>
> In contrast to this shining and easy childhood that brought forth an upright and noble character, an autobiographical note in the preface to his Qianjin fang 千金方(Priceless Prescriptions) notes that he was a rather sickly boy who underwent all kinds of treatments, thus inspiring a great interest in medical matters and an inclination toward longevity practices and Daoist seclusion."

> By Livia Kohn, ´A Sourcebook in Chinese Longevity.´

Sun Simiao wrote the following verses on seasonal breathing practices contained in the Xiuzhen shishu. This is his advice on how to align oneself with the rhythm of nature.

> In spring, breathe xu for clear eyes and so wood can aid your liver.
>
> In summer, reach for he, so that heart and fire can be at peace.
>
> In fall, breathe si to stabilize and gather metal, keeping the lungs moist.
>
> For the kidneys, next, breathe chui and see your inner water calm.
>
> The triple heater needs your xi to expel all heat and troubles.
>
> In all four seasons take long breaths, so spleen can process food.
>
> And, of course, avoid exhaling noisily, not letting even your ears hear it.
>
> This practice is most excellent and will help preserve your divine elixir.
>
> -from the *Daoist Canon*

He wrote extensively on living a life based on moderation in all things, including diet and the bedchamber, physical exercises as the foundation for guiding chi, and self massage, 'anmo', as a daily practice. In Sun Simiao's written works, regular daily exercises play a crucial role in both healing and long life chi cultivation. A healthy body supports the quest for long life and prepares one for the higher stages of immortality practice. Some of his advice reflected the cultural taboos of the time, but most held sound practical advice for a balanced healthy life.

The role of healing exercises is also found in the work of the other major figure in Tang longevity techniques, Sima Chengzhen, (647-735). A native of Henan, he was a descendant of the imperial house of the Jin dynasty that ruled China in the third and fourth centuries. Trained well in the classics and arts of the gentleman, such as calligraphy and poetry, Sima is described as a highly precocious and very intelligent child.

Still, rather than dedicating himself to standard Confucian service, he opted for a career in Daoism, which in the eighth century had risen to official status and was the main religion as supported by the state. He began his Daoist studies on Mount Song, the central of the five sacred mountains located near Luoyang in his native Henan. At the age of 21, in 669, he underwent Daoist ordination under Pan Shizheng, the eleventh patriarch of Highest Clarity. Continuing his climb through the Daoist hierarchy and absorbing all the esoteric rites and scriptures of the different schools, Sima was chosen to succeed his teacher as twelfth patriarch in 684.

Sima Chengzhen was invited to court four times, first by Empress Wu, the same woman who tried to capture Ho Hsien Ku and bring her to court to teach the empress immortality practices.

Like Sun Simiao, he traveled widely, propagating Daoist teachings and seeking out learned masters. He was well versed in medical knowledge and engaged in the various longevity practices, abstaining from grains for extended periods, taking herbal medicines to enhance and transform his *qi*, and undertaking physical and breathing exercises. However, unlike

Sun Simiao who had a predominantly medical focus, Sima's entire practice was steeped in the spiritual dimension of the teaching. He became known for his extraordinary powers.

Sima lived a long and healthy life. In June of 735, after announcing his imminent transformation for transfer to an official post in the celestial administration, he sat quietly in meditation and accompanied by white cranes, purple clouds, and celestial music, ascended to emptiness, vanishing before the astounded eyes of his disciples (Engelhardt 1987, 51). The Daoist master thus returned to his true home above the clouds. Sima recommended the absorption of solar energies for healing. To treat ailments practice right after sunrise and preferably when the weather is calm and mild. Sit up straight, face the sun, close your eyes, curl the hands into fists, and click the teeth nine times. Then visualize the scarlet brilliance and purple rays of the sun, pull them into the body as you inhale, and swallow them. Envision this healing energy entering the inner organ or area of the body that is afflicted by the ailment. One needs to purify the *qi* through the gradual elimination of ordinary food and instead ingest herbal concoctions and celestial energies.

To make sure that the *qi* reaches all the different parts of the body, practitioners actively visualize it moving into all its parts. Absorbing sunlight in the morning, First, visualize the *qi* in the lungs for some time, then feel it run along the shoulders and into the arms, until it reaches your hands that have been curled into fists. After this envision it gently moving down from the lungs and into the stomach and spleen area, from where it moves into the kidneys. Allow it to flow through the thighs into the legs and feet. You will know that you are doing it right when you feel a slight tingling between skin and flesh, sort of like the crawling of tiny insects.

*To summarize:* For both major representatives of the tradition in the Tang dynasty, Sun Simiao and Sima Chengzhen, the ultimate goal of Daoist practices is the complete overcoming of worldly attachments and the final attainment of immorality, a spiritual state of otherworldly residence.

Healing exercises play an important part and appear in various levels of the immortal curriculum, but they are secondary to visualizations, *qi*-absorptions, and ecstatic excursions.

In many ways the methods the Tang masters adopted continue the tradition of Highest Clarity, the dominant school of Daoism at the time. Yet they are also very medically aware and make health and wholeness an important part of the process. For the first time in Chinese history they consciously integrate healing, longevity, and immortality into a complete Daoist system of self-realization and spiritual attainment.

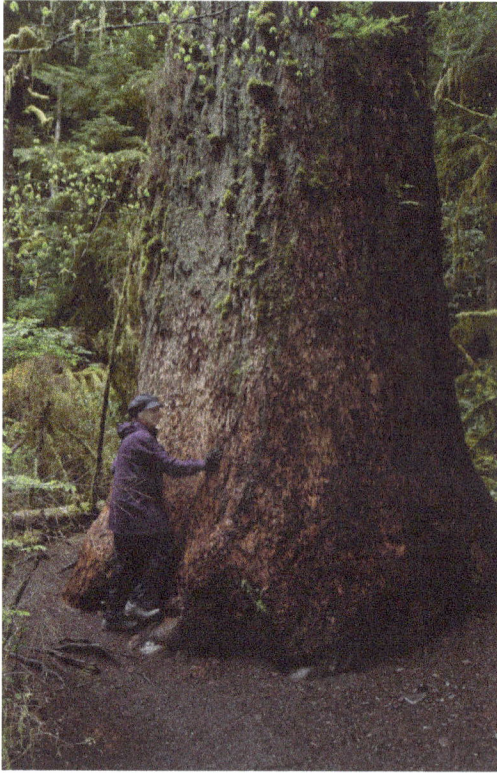

Author in the Olympic National Forest

# Exchanging Chi with Trees

Taoist tree meditations connect you energetically to a forest or to a specific tree with the intention of circulating your chi for physical and emotional healing. As you learn to circulate chi between yourself and a tree many thoughts and emotions may arise. You may choose to sit or stand quietly and absorb the essence of a particular tree, allowing for deep stirrings of intuition to arise within you. Or you may set a specific intention to commune with the tree, sensing into its flow and color. You can extend your open palms toward a tree and begin to feel its vibration, even sense into a subtle movement. Soon you realize that trees are not solitary beings, they are connected to everything around them, above them and below them. The sun moon and stars, the air, rain, clouds, wind, the soil and fungi, the creatures in the air and on the land are in relationship to the tree. Trees have personalities just like people, of varying shapes, sizes, qualities and contributions to nature and all life. Maybe you have a favorite tree that you remember from childhood. There are trees in towns and cities, forests and near rivers that I recall with great fondness for their rightness of being and of the beauty that they contribute to the place. The Wood element in TCM engenders the higher virtues of expansion, growth and generosity. These virtues are easily seen in the patient, yet tenacious, life force of a tree.

Once a tree has chosen you, or you have decided upon a tree to meditate with, move into the energetic chi field of the tree. Open yourself and the palms of your hands to sense the aura of the tree, and step slowly forward to a comfortable distance. Begin breathing with the intention of absorbing essence of the tree and all nature around you; inhale through your nose and from every pore in your body, exhale from your mouth release toxins from every pore in your body. Trees are masters at transforming chi from sun and the atmosphere. Conclude your tree meditation by leaning your spine up against the tree for a few minutes.

Trees emit color just as people produce color in their auras. Today I felt/saw a large Douglas fir tree present the color yellow to me, so I received this color to assist my Earth element to come into harmony. Master Wang Liping has this to say about trees and color: Pine trees emit green which relates to Wood element and the liver, Cedar trees emit red with relates to the Fire element and the heart, Willow trees emit yellow for the Earth element and stomach, Poplar tree give off a White color which is represented by the Metal element and the Lungs, Cypress trees emit a dark blue/black color which represents the Water element and assists the kidneys. Some people see or sense color, others may feel color. However you have developed your senses is good, and there are many trees in the world, so have some fun in finding what each of them has to teach you.

Another method of working with tree medicine is to circulate your chi out of the soles of your feet into the roots of the tree, and then bringing in tree energy to the crown of your head from the top of the tree. Slow down your respiration to match nature and the tree that you are connected with.

Today as I was getting to know a specific tree in the forest near my home, I sensed a stillness in it's life force and that brought me to the realization of the Stillness and the Tao. Stillness is not simply the lack of movement, but the deep un-manifested creative force which gives birth to the balance of yin and yang. Of course a tree moves as it grows, but very slowly and in keeping with right timing.

Like each of us, trees make contributions to all life as an integrated unified field of life. It is food for thought as we ponder our own contributions to life. We may not be as famous as the giant Redwoods of California, or Tane Mahuta, (lord of the forest) revered by the Maori of New Zealand, but we are important in our individual contribution to the evolution of our own destiny and consciousness. It is this refined consciousness which engenders immortality.

# Eating or not eating: Bigu/Fasting

Bigu, or fasting, is an immortality practice which supports in the transformation of the physical body into a vehicle of pure Dao, independent of food and drink and living on *qi* alone. I was told a story a few years ago by a priest who grew up at Wudan Mountain. A woman who lived at Wudan mountain in China never ate, but went daily to sweep the steps of every shrine and temple. There she would prostrate herself and touch her forehead to the floor. She lived a pure and simple life. When it became known to the outside world that she was not eating, the reporters flooded in to the temple to see her. This outer distraction broke the focus of her contemplative practice and she was no longer able to maintain her fasting. This is our dilemma today. How do we maintain focus with our practices without being distracted by the outer world?

There are records of the gradual process that the physical body went through in the first few weeks of fasting; the changes in the complexion of the skin, the physical weakness, the lessening of bowel activity. Eventually the body and spirit are light and can fly on the clouds like the immortals. The steps toward total fasting included eating only grains, then only vegetables, then no food after noon, drinking water with talismans and mineral essences, absorbing chi from the directions, the sun, moon and stars, absorbing primordial qi and cosmic energy to merge with heaven and earth, and finally embryo respiration, breathing the pure qi of creation, to become one with the Dao. The initial response of the body to fasting is detoxification and the feeling of weakness. After several months of fasting, breathing practice, herbal formulas and guiding chi the practitioner begins to feel strong and cheerful. The third step in the Fusion of the Five elements meditation practice is useful to mention here. It is Sealing the senses; quieting the internal organs to overcome external temptation and distraction by drawing awareness inward. I have done this meditation practice; it is very calming and is best done away from any distractions. The Daoist term for retreat is *biquan,* which means closed gate.

Traditionally, one would begin with the absorption of *qi* at sunrise in a special cave set up for the practice. The process required a gradual adjustment, over a period of about six weeks. The practitioner needed to purify their *qi* through the gradual elimination of ordinary food with the replacement of herbal concoctions and celestial energies. Simply not eating is no guarantee that the fasting will result in energy transformation. One must be able to absorb and circulate chi, replacing external nourishment with internal nourishment. Listening inward is the precondition for fasting practices which lead to chi transformation.

We have an excellent guidepost in Sun Bu'ers poetry as apparently this is the practice she adopted to become immortal.

"Cultivation is like a huge smelting operation
One can turn things into a mountain or lake.
The process builds upon a passion for transformation.
In the morning, eat the qi of the sun, like a turtle,
In the evening, absorb the essence of the moon, like a toad.
Gathering elixir astutely, the body feels light and lighter.
And when the original spirit visits

Ten thousand apertures emit a bright clear radiance."
Translation of poem 10 by Jill Gonet.

In our Western way of thinking, fasting or light eating is recommended during an illness such as a cold. Chinese tradition would be to offer the patient a thin soup or congee which is easily digested. We know now that short periods of fasting stimulates the immune system and with proper attention to the body, fasting may support health and recovery from disease. A simple way to create a personal ritual around cosmic changes is to eat only fruit and water on the new moon and the full moon each month. This is a practice in some Daoist temples. Another practice that you might like to try is exchanging chi with nature; something like the tree meditation practice, but on a larger scale. Allow the chi of nature to enter into your organs. This brings balance and peace to the body and spirit. When you fast it is not to starve yourself, but to understand yourself at a deeper level. Know where your weak spots are and allow weak or diseased cells to be destroyed and replaced by new cells.

Using herbs as food has a long history in China. One group of herbs was called food herbs, eaten for general nourishment. The Daoist hermits called these herbs *immortal foods* and explained that they could rejuvenate health and prolong life. One such herb was pyrrosia, or tongue fern. Herbs were often used as the main part of their diet along with fruits and nuts and seeds. The other groups of herbs were considered medicinal herbs which were dispensed by a medical professional. Formulas used during fasting regimes might include minerals and fungi that would be found naturally occurring in the mountains; such as mica, pine tree sap and needles, mushrooms, the roots of plants like asparagus, and lyceum (goji berries). Chinese people were used to eating these types of foods in times of famine, so they were familiar with the tonifying quality of them. Ho Hsien Ku, the female immortal, was said to eat Mica on her long forays into the mountains. Foods, herbs, plants and minerals that we eat have spirit and chi that are transformed into our body.

Swallowing chi and saliva is a common Daoist practice; as one progresses with internal alchemy the saliva becomes as sweet as dew. There are specific instructions on how and when to swallow chi; it goes like this. Inhale through the nose and hold your breath in the mouth to form a mixture of saliva and the inhaled chi of your breath. Circle your tongue between the lips and the outside of the teeth 36 times and swish the saliva around in your mouth before swallowing the saliva. Swallow 3 times and direct the saliva into the cauldron of the lower tan tien. Do this as many times a day as you are able and guide the chi with your hands by rubbing them down the front of your body, from throat to belly. Here you are replacing food in the body with chi.

Daoist immortal sage Chen Tuan spoke about swallowing saliva in his Four Season Qigong instructions. See "Chen Tuan's Four Season Internal Kung Fu", by Stuart Alve Olson.

Once the Daoist practitioner has given up food and is entirely ingesting or living on chi, she has retreated from society and practices specific breathing techniques and chi guiding to perfect and sustain her immortal body. Advanced practices such as this require that the adept be completely immersed in the realm of spirit and not have contact of any kind with others. This allows the practitioner to conserve highly refined chi which is used for internal alchemical practice and spiritual attainment.

Preparation leading to this advanced practice may take years and a clear focus. As the physical body becomes lighter and freer, the adept returns to a primordial state of being like an embryo; now supported by the universe rather than the womb. The movement of the Dao is returning and many Daoist practices have this focus of returning to original primordial chi. As a lineage practice you can say that Daoist practices remind you and lead you in a full circle of beginning and completion, to the knowing of yourself as being one with the infinite and immortal creation.

# I Ching

The I Ching: Book of Change is a book of Symbols and Numbers which gives us advice on the right timing for any action to be accomplished with the least amount of effort. Everything in the universe is seeking harmony and balance. As a trusted advisor the I Ching can guide us in all of the situations we encounter in life. Consulting the I Ching is a Science when one understands the symbols and numbers which create the structure, and an Art when divined with your intuition. We all create our own reality based on our life experiences and beliefs. The I Ching provides us with information on how to avoid misfortune by using the right attitude and the right timing. Our fate or destiny depends on our actions. Good decisions create harmony and balance. A woman's life is filled with decisions which affect her and those around her in numerous ways. Having a trusted advisor in times of transition can ease the process of change and bring a peace of mind and spirit that benefits everyone in your home and community. The I Ching can help you to develop a deep trust in the rhythm of life, and in all nature. The six lines of each hexagram in the I Ching bring us to completion in our actions and guide us to "not overdo" things, but rather to simplify. The 7th line, if it were to be visible, would indicate excess in our actions. We can use it as a resting point, just as the universe rested on the 7th day. Seven might symbolize non action and surrender to the wisdom of the Dao.

Named YiJing in China, it is the Book of Change, or Wu Shu; Shamans book (shu meaning calculation). What kind of Change is the I Ching suggesting? The progress of the 64 hexagrams is gradual, organic and wavelike in pattern. Everything is in a continuous process of change in the universe, and that includes our lives. There is a short wavelike process happening from one hexagram to the next, and a longer wavelike process going on from on group to another, and from beginning to end. No change is straight and smooth, change is a process. If we can harmonize our lives with nature, then our progression will be a smooth evolutionary pattern of change, rather than a sharp dramatic shift up and down.

*Live within the laws of nature and the laws of human affairs.*

Fu Xi (an ancient Chinese shaman) saw a pattern which he called He Tu, or river pattern. This pattern has evolved in the 8000 years since he recorded it and represents the phenomenon of the universe forming. The He Tu gave birth to the symbols and numbers which later evolved to become the trigrams which comprise the 64 hexagrams that we study today. "He Tu", the name of this map, was seen by Fu Xi in a pattern which formed on the side of a water horse that emerged from the Yellow river. The dots of the He Tu pattern were transformed into lines many years later by Shao Yong. (a.d. 1011-1077) He also assigned numbers to the lines and this became the Earlier Heaven arrangement of the Bagua.

For over 5000 years the information of the He Tu and LuoShu patterns traveled with nomads, seers, shaman and fortunetellers who used the patterns as a weather and star chart, as system of magic and prediction. Recorded on oracle bones, shells, jade and possibly animal hides, the He Tu and LuoShu patterns of Fu Xi survived due to the accurate and potent information that was held in these supernatural designs.

The I Ching divination system was developed before Chinese characters were invented. The original I Ching text was composed of only trigrams ( 3 horizontal lines) and had no written language. One had to master the symbolic meanings of the trigrams to do a good job in divination. The images of the trigrams and hexagrams would be displayed in the home as a guiding image, called the Fastening Text. The text was fastened under the symbol of a chosen trigram, (8 trigrams which represent the eight forces of nature), to show its significance.

*The purpose of the I Ching is to influence Humans to become superior persons, and to benefit others like mother earth does.*

### Symbols
You are probably familiar with the 3 lines that make up a pattern which is arranged in a circle, called a Bagua, or 8 sided symbol. There are 8 trigrams that combine to make the 64 hexagrams of the I Ching. The 8 trigrams represent the 8 forces of Nature which evolved as an integral concept in the philosophy of Daoism.

Trigrams have attributes like humans have personalities. Some of the attributes of the trigrams are listed below.

### Heaven; Qian
Pure yang; creative energy of the universe. Not literally heaven or the universe, but Qian brings things into being. It is active and initiating. Male

### Earth; Kun
Pure Yin; responsive energy of the universe. Resembles earth but it is not earth. Heaven and earth complement each other

and cannot manifest alone. Kun is passive and receptive. Female.

## Fire; Li

Heat and light. Brightness. Symbolizes intelligence and wisdom. Distinction between right and wrong.

## Water; Kan

Symbol of danger or difficulty. Darkness. Represents the moon. Gentle power.

## Thunder; Zhen

Arousing energy in the universe; creative energy. Triggers things to grow and take action once they have been created. Agitates, awakens, inspires, uplifts, elevates and exalts.

## Wind; Xun

Sometimes called wood, represents a proceeding, penetrating energy; the wind blowing over the earth and the tree penetrating into the ground. Proceed gently. A gentle breeze with bright sun or mild rain is the best weather. It never violates and is therefore easily accepted.

## Mountain; Gen

Soothing energy that provides a structure. It stops things from growing or advancing. Calms things down, holds them back and keeps them within bounds, or even to a standstill. The symbol of meditation

## Lake; Dui

Exhilarating energy in the universe. Radiates cheerfulness and joy to stimulate growth.

There are several methods of divination or prediction which bring you to a hexagram or a trigram. Here I offer you some insight into the symbolic meaning of the trigrams, which make up hexagrams.

Trigrams have a natural movement, as do the seasons. 4 of the Trigrams are Yang and move up toward heaven, and 4 are Yin, moving down toward earth.

Each hexagram has an inner spirit and an outer presence. All of the 64 hexagrams are created from two trigrams stacked upon each other, ( six lines arranged horizontally) and there are two trigrams couched inside of the hexagram. Called the inner trigrams, or the nucleus, we glean the inner meaning of the hexagram. Now we have 4 symbols to work with as we interpret our divination. There is an inner spirit which reflects our inner motivation and an outer presence which reflects the outer situation.

Lines 2,3,4 create the lower inner trigram. Lines 3,4,5 create the top inner trigram. When you extract these two inner trigrams and stack them you get a new hexagram; this inner recipe has a new essence and a new meaning to contemplate. Just as different molecules form to create specific substances, the trigrams combine to create the hexagrams.

**Suggestions to think about when looking at the overall pattern of I Ching.**
If you look at King Wen's (12th century BC.) arrangement of the 64 hexagrams (later heaven arrangement) found in most books you will see patterns emerge. The I Ching, Book of Change, begins with pure heaven and pure earth hexagrams,

(hexagrams 1 and 2), but we do not see heaven or earth trigrams in the last 18 hexagrams of the total 64. If the progression of the 64 hexagrams symbolize the story of our life, or the progression in any project, then what is the message here? Beginnings require focus, energy, yang perseverance and clear intentions, like the Heaven over Heaven trigram of the first hexagram. Looking at the pattern or trigrams in the last 18 of the 64 will tell us that another type of focus is required to complete cycles and projects, and a life.

As we know there is a long tradition of Alchemy in Daoist practices. Indeed, the lines of the hexagrams represent the 6 steps in alchemical reactions. Many advanced Daoist meditation practices use fire and water to create internal alchemy, (Nei Dan), in our bodies for purification. The last 2 hexagrams of the I Ching are pure combinations of fire and water trigrams. Does this indicate that at the end of life, or the end of a cycle we must purify and dissolve? Please study the trigrams and the hexagrams for they appear in an order which will give you advice. Clear your mind and open your heart of the guidance that is offered.

I Ching has two parts; An upper canon with 30 hexagrams. #1 heaven# 2 earth #29 water #30 fire. These four hexagrams are the 4 cardinal directions of the pre heaven bagua. The upper canon represents the Dao of heaven. The lower canon has 34 hexagrams which represent the Dao of humanity, ending with hexagrams #63 and #64, a blending of fire and water trigrams.
The I Ching summarizes all phenomena in the universe in the 64 hexagrams. The hexagram represents the phenomena and the 6 lines represent the stages of change. So, phenomena develop in 6 stages. When any situation reaches the 7th stage

things change dramatically; the old vanishes and something new appears. When things are taken to the extreme they revert to the beginning.

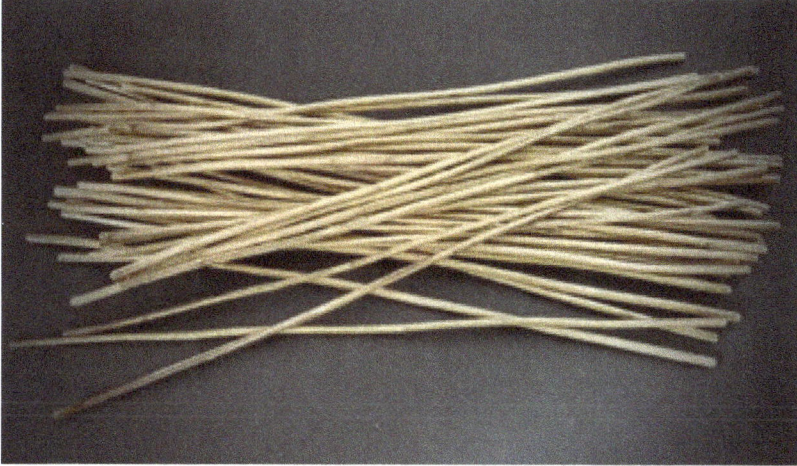

Yarrow sticks

**The lines of the hexagram are like a recipe**
Line 6 passes the peak, or done in excess, goes into next situation
Line 5 is the culmination of the situation
Line 4 is the resolution, it transcends the obstacle or conflict
Line 3 represents a problem or obstacle
Line 2 is the character of the situation, observe the situation
Line 1 is the beginning of the situation

**Numbers**
To the ancient Chinese, numbers were alive and mysterious. They symbolized the ceaseless motion between heaven and

earth. Odd numbers were yang, even numbers were considered yin.

The numbers 3 and 5 embody the way of the universe.

The universe is constructed of 3 layers in space and time. In space the layers are upper, tian heaven, lower kun earth, and middle layer ren, humanity. In time the layers are past present and future. Human beings are a microcosm reflecting the macrocosm. Human beings are constructed of 3 layers, jing, chi and shen.

Five is the number of the directions. Four cardinal directions with you in the middle or central place, making 5. Five is seen as the Ancient symbol of the shaman, or a builders square.

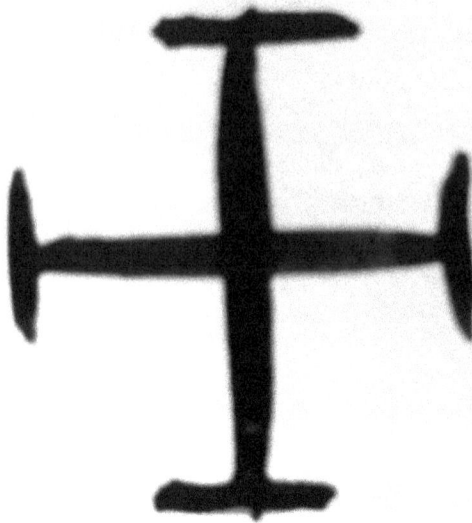

There is a transition from a number to a gua (trigram). If you are using coins to cast the hexagram you assign a value to the head or tail of the coin as such: a Yin line has the value 8. A Yang line has the value 7. The values of 7 and 8 are unchanging lines. 6 and 9 are moving lines and will yield a second hexagram.

_____          _____  _____

Yang Line                    Yin Line

*Time line*

6000 BC Fuxi sees He Tu and LuoShu patterns

2000 BC first written record of the I Ching

1000 BC Duke of Zhao comments on In Ching

1050 BC King Wen arranges the hexagram into Later heaven sequence and writes commentary on the hexagrams

500 BC Confucius comments on the I Ching (creating the moral and reason school)

1100 AD Shao Yong arranges Early Heaven sequence from He Tu pattern, and translates the numbers into lines of the yao; trigrams.

18th century. Using 0 and 1, a German mathematician creates the Binary system of counting and sees that this information already exists in the 64 hexagrams of I Ching, and in the work of Shao Yong.

1987 international symposium on Zhou I analysis showed the Lo Shu and He Tu to be 3 dimensional meteorological maps and star compass and climate chart.

He Tu; River pattern

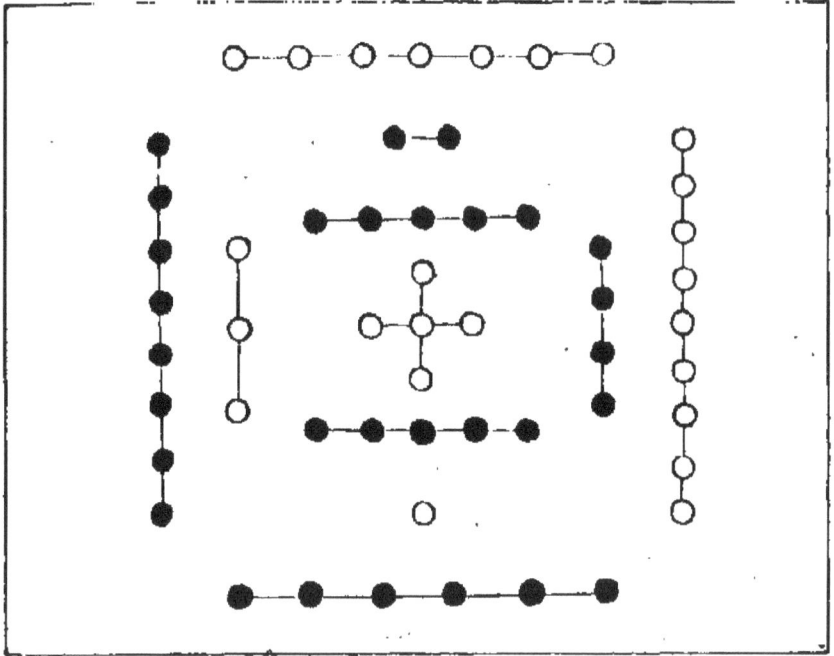

*The Chinese believe that number is related to destiny. When you are conceived you have a destined number. This applies to objects also.*

Our lives consist of cycles within cycles. ANY CYCLE THAT WE SET IN MOTION CONTAINS ALL THE HEXAGRAMS. SO, FINISH EACH CYCLE, IN A GOOD MOOD. This releases the energy. Like falling asleep, or dying, a cycle ends. Finish EACH day in a good mood. Finish your life in a good mood with all projects completed.

**Casting the I Ching**

There are several ways to cast the I Ching; using 3 coins, 50 yarrow sticks, the reduction of 3 numbers, and using the palm of one's hand. Whichever way you choose to study and use for divination or prediction, it is important to bring the right attitude into your space and to phrase your question with a clear intention to receive guidance.

*Asking your question*
Slow down and observe. Feel the energetic connection of the symbols and words that you use to interpret them. In the greater universe individual changes are relatively unimportant, it is the PROCESS of change itself which needs to be emphasized. In other words, the quality of chi that you bring to the process of change is very important.

*The Casting of Yarrow Sticks for Divining of I Ching*

Hold 50 yarrow stalks in your left hand

Put one aside, this one symbolizes the commencement of Tai Chi (ultimate beginning) from the void; the state before heaven and earth differentiated.
1. Divide the remaining 49 at random into 2 bunches, hold one bunch in each hand. The left represents Heaven, the right Earth.
2. Take one stalk from the right hand and put it between the pinky and ring finger of the left hand. This represents Humanity.
3. Take 4 stalks at a time from the left hand bundle and put them aside until there are 4 or less remaining the hand Place these remaining stalks between the ring finger and the middle finger of your left hand.

4. Take 4 stalks at a time from your right hand bundle and put them aside until there are 4 or less remaining in your hand. Place the remaining stalks between the middle and index finger of your left hand.
5. Collect all the stalks in your left hand and add them up. The sum should be either 5 or 9. (the first time only)

Set these aside (as a visual counter) and repeat steps 1-5 two more times with the remaining stalks. THIS PROCESS PRODUCES ONE LINE; THE BOTTOM LINE OF THE HEXAGRAM.

After you have done this 3 times, you are holding one last bundle of stalks to be counted. Set down 4 at a time and count the number of bundles that you have; 6,7,8 or 9. Do this 5 more times to create the entire hexagram of 6 lines. Build the hexagram from bottom to top.

**Casting the I Ching with Coins**
Number values equal a line. This method creates hexagrams using 3 coins. Tails have a value of 3 heads a value of 2. Toss the 3 coins once to create a line. Repeat 6 times to create a hexagram. the first toss is the bottom line of the hexagram. Build up from there

| | COINS |
|---|---|
| 6 __ __ changes to 7 _____ | 6 3 heads |
| 7_____ not changing | 7 2 heads 1 tail |
| 8__ __ not changing | 8 2 tails 1 head |
| 9_____ changes to 8 __ __ | 9 3 tails |

Changing Lines create a second hexagram, so you have two hexagrams to consider. And you also have the inner, or nuclear trigrams to consider. This is a lot of information, so take your time to digest it and see how it guides you.

I hope you will enjoy your study of the I Ching, Book of Change. Find a book that you like and take your time in understanding the complexity of this ancient system of divination. I enjoy the writing of Alfred Huang, "The Complete I Ching." And if you are looking for a way to learn how to make a prediction based on the reduction of 3 digit numbers I recommend Master Zhongxian Wu, "Seeking the Spirit of the Book of Change."

# Fusion of the 5 Elements

Fusion of the 5 Elements is a Daoist meditation which utilizes several elements of your foundation practices; inner smile, six healing sounds, microcosmic orbit. Also, you will rely on an understanding of the 5 elements and the emotions attached to them, and the 8 forces of nature as defined by the 8 trigrams. The unique geometry of the Bagua and 8 trigrams creates a visual vortex of chi. Up until now you have developed a high quality and quantity of Chi with your qigong and meditation practices, the thoughts you have, the emotions you feel, the foods your eat, the air you breathe, even the amount of your sleep. It takes a high quality and quantity of Chi (energy) to be successful when you attempt energy practices such as Fusion of the 5 elements.

After many years of study and practice with masters in the mountains of China, Yi Eng (Yi Eng, or I Yun, means White Cloud) taught this practice to my teacher, Mantak Chia. There is no initiation or ceremony involved in these practices, simply Practice. As you practice you set up a foundation for your next steps. If you are prepared in basic practices of any kind, the next steps will come easily and naturally.

Fusion of the five elements Part I includes 9 inner alchemy Formulas of internal spiritual cultivation that were given to us by White Cloud; Yi Eng. Many generations of Daoist Masters refined their experiences into nine stages of inner alchemy. White Cloud lived in China to be 96. I estimate that he passed on in 1977.

The goal of Fusion inner alchemy formulas is to refine our consciousness by fusing and harmonizing our physical and energetic bodies for the experience of immortality.

The 9 formulas enhance the wisdom of the I Ching which teaches us to refine our Chi so that we use the right timing and correct attitude to approach life, enabling humans to leave the body without desires or attachments in the physical world. We thus reconnect to Primordial Chi.

To become fully aware of our primordial self we must first purify the organs and emotions of the physical body. We practice inner smile and 6 healings sounds to help us along this path. Bone breathing qigong and Chi Nei Tsang abdominal massage is also vital to bring the body into a high state of preparedness for these alchemical practices. If your prenatal chi is weak in one area of the 5 elements, then Fusion of the 5 elements will balance you in a harmonious way and allow pure virtue to shine from every cell in your body.

Using the 8 forces of nature, which are represented by the 8 trigrams used in I Ching, (Heaven, Earth, Fire, Water, Lake, Thunder, Mountain and Wind), we create an 8 sided structure, named the Bagua (Pakua), as a three dimensional energy vortex to magnetize pure Universal Chi which transforms and neutralizes any negative emotions held in the cells of our organs. Once the Chi is transformed in to pure original source chi it is gathered into a Cauldron which we locate in the lower tan tien, (sea of chi) below the navel. Just as you did with the Microcosmic Orbit meditation, you will gather chi into the cauldron to create a Radiant Pearl of refined, compressed chi. This energy pearl is used to transfer consciousness and is circulated through meridians and later returned to the Cauldron in the lower tan tien to become a spiritual embryo. We strive to keep the cauldron full so that our overall level of chi is a dynamic reservoir of health.

All levels of Fusion practices will purify the organs of the body. When this is accomplished, the mind is much clearer as it is receiving a high quality of chi information from the internal organs. Seek the guidance of an instructor who has substantial experience with this practice, to assist you in attaining realistic goals.

**9 Formulas of Fusion of the five elements Part I**
In part 1 your goal is to develop awareness of the pearl that you create in your lower tan tien and to transform negative emotions so that the organs are vibrant with original chi.

*Part 1 Formulas 1-5*
1. Create a cauldron in your lower tan tien. Create 4 pakuas to transform chi and a pearl in the cauldron to store, or circulate chi.
2. Spiral negative or imbalanced chi (chi that is too hot or too cold) from each of the organs to be transformed into collection spheres, which are the same color as the associated organ, outside of the body.
3. Sealing the senses; quieting the internal organs to overcome external temptation and distraction by drawing awareness inward.
4. Transforming the emotions by spiraling them into collections spheres to be transformed into pure useable chi in the cauldron.
5. Pearl is projected and formed into an energy body.

*Part 2 Formulas 6-9*

6. Create a virgin boy and girl; using the images of children to give form to pure energy.
7. Totem animals as protection; using the images of animals to defend the organs.
8. Planets and stars as protection and empowerment.
9. Transfer consciousness to the energy body.

There are Advanced Fusion practices, (that will not be introduced completely here) known as the Enlightenment of Kan and Li. When the Fire of the Heart combines with the Water of the Kidneys there is a reuniting with the Primordial Force. This process of water over fire (hexagram 63 in the I Ching) creates a steaming in the cauldron of the tan tien. The steaming cleanses, purifies and strengthens the organs, meridians, lymph and brain. Internal Alchemy follows the same principles, or formulas, that we find in the natural world, the I Ching, and the science of cooking; Use the right amount of chi and the correct time to get the best result.

Solstices and Equinoxes are auspicious times to practice as the Earth energies are aligned with other planets and moons and Suns in the universe. Spring Equinox is a time of balance in yin and yang, light and dark, heat and cold. Summer Solstice in the northern hemisphere is a time of long day and short night. Where I live currently in Bellingham Washington, the sun rises at 5am and sets at 9:15pm. There is still light until 10pm. The rising Yang energy of the morning is a great time to practice. It is important, however, to keep your yang fire chi from escaping too much in the long hot days of summer. The opposite is true here in the Winter; very long nights which are great for Yin Water practice to soothe the kidneys. Step 3 of fusion is great in Winter.

**The Beginning Practice**

To begin your Fusion of the 5 elements practice we will do step 1. In your mind's eye picture a cauldron forming in your lower tan tien. This will hold the chi that you bring in through the pakua's to form the pearl. Create it however you like to see it. I am going to guide you in steps 1,2 and 4 in this section as I have found them to be extremely cohesive and beneficial.

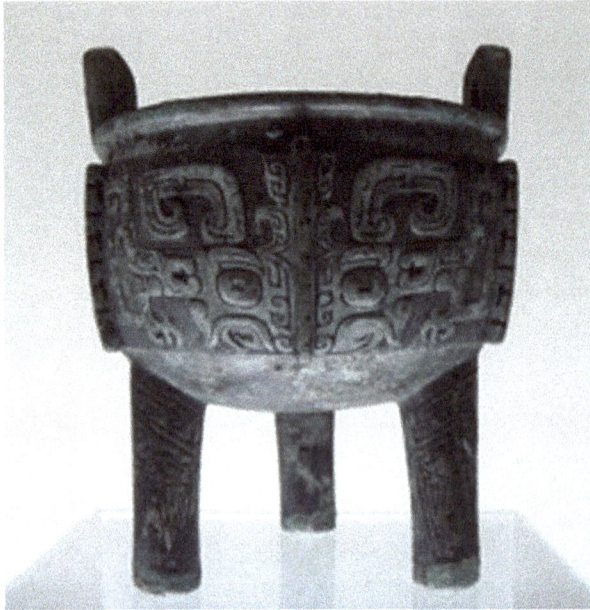

Next create 4 pakuas which look like a vortex of moving energy. One on the front of your body, one on the back, and one on the right and left sides of your body. These connect into the cauldron in your lower tan tien. Each pakua has all 8 trigrams, forces of nature, around the edges of the vortex.

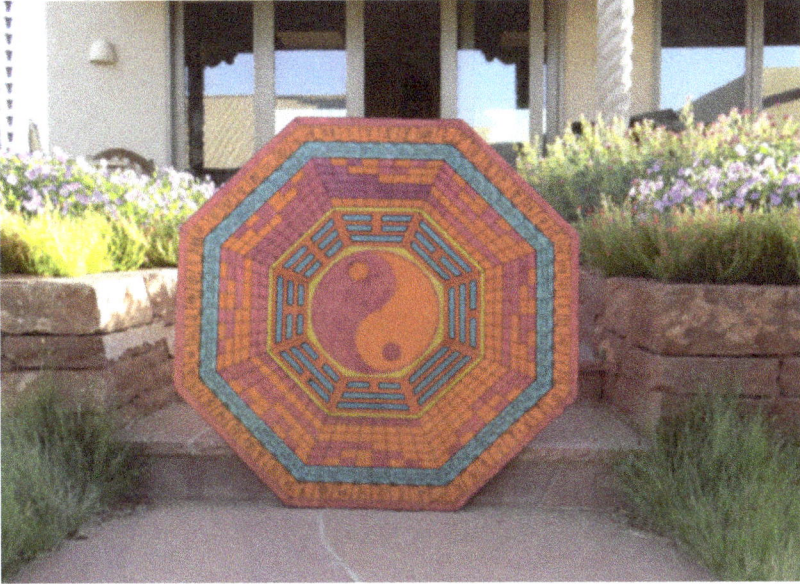

Spin the pakua in a clockwise direction and gather in pure chi from the beginning of the universe. Let it gather and condense in the cauldron to form a pearl.

2. Spiral negative or imbalanced chi (chi that is too hot or too cold) from each of the organs to be transformed into collection spheres, which are the same color as the associated organ, outside of the body.

4. Transforming the emotions by spiraling them into collections spheres to be transformed into pure useable chi in the cauldron.

Create the collection spheres

Imagine in your mind's eye an empty red sphere in 6 inches front of your heart and an empty blue sphere near the perineum and bladder.

Spiral out negative emotions and excess heat or cold

Spiral out from the heart and small intestines any imbalanced chi or negative emotions that are hanging out in the organs. Release this chi into the sphere.

Into the blue collection sphere spiral out from the kidneys and bladder any negative emotions or chi that is too cold. Release chi to be transformed into the sphere.

Transform chi into pure source chi in the cauldron

Now spin the front Pakua very fast in a clockwise rotation and gather in the two spheres (red and blue) into the moving vortex. As the chi is suctioned into and through the pakua it is transformed and elevated into pure source chi which now flows into the cauldron. Take a moment and feel the freedom and lightness in your body and the gathering chi in the cauldron.

Create the collection spheres

Next create an empty green collection sphere to the right of your body near the liver, and an empty white collection sphere to the left side of your body.

Spiral out negative emotions and excess dampness or dryness

Release any negative emotions from the liver and gallbladder, and any excess dampness into the green collection sphere.

Release all negative emotions or excess dryness from the lungs and large intestine into the white collection sphere.

Transform chi into pure source chi in the cauldron

Again, spin the front Pakua very fast in a clockwise rotation and gather in the two spheres (green and white) into the moving vortex. As the chi is suctioned into and through the pakua it is transformed and elevated into pure source chi which now flows into the cauldron. Take a moment and feel the freedom and lightness in your body and the gathering chi in the cauldron.

Create the final collection sphere

Visualize a golden yellow collection sphere about 6 inches in front of your solar plexus near the stomach and pancreas.
From the stomach and pancreas spiral out negative emotions; whatever takes you out of balance, and any chi that is too hot or too cold.

Transform chi into pure source chi in the cauldron

Spin the front Pakua very fast in a clockwise rotation and gather in the final sphere (yellow) into the moving vortex. As the chi is suctioned into and through the pakua it is transformed and elevated into pure source chi which now flows into the cauldron. Take a moment and feel the freedom and lightness in your body and the gathering chi in the cauldron.

Now that you have cleared all internal the organ's chi you can focus your mind's eye on the cauldron. Watch and feel as the pure transformed chi condenses into a luminous pearl. This pearl of chi is now available to circulate in the Microcosmic orbit, or can be stored in the lower tan tien as your personal source of chi and power to be used for health and intuition.

Fusion practice can be done as often as you need to transform chi and stay in a neutral balanced place in your life.

# Jing chi and shen

Imagine a candle burning brightly. The candle wax is your body's physical jing, the flame is your breath, vitality, chi and the shen is the light of your spirit. As you refine and cultivate physical health you are creating a foundation which connects jing to chi. As you regulate your breathing in meditation and qigong your chi connects with shen. As you cultivate virtue and awareness in daily living, becoming more conscious, you connect your shen to the un-manifest void and your immortal soul.

Cultivating the Three Treasures form the trunk for the yang sheng, (long life), tree of nurturing life. The branches are your jing, chi and shen. The roots are the philosophical principles of the Tao, yin and yang, and 5 elements creation theory. Longevity is the fruit of your practice. Tranquility is the result of practice, and the gateway to immortality which allows shen (spirit) to return to the void/Dao.

*Qi is the bridge between matter and spirit.*

Longevity, Yang Shen, is an enlightened attitude towards self and nature that can lead to a harmonious way of living. Guard your Three Treasures to find balance and harmony in this life. Harmony in the human body is based on the functioning of Jing, Chi and Shen; or the 3 Treasures. Harmony in nature is seen in the unending relationship between the sun, moon and stars.

Qi is vibrating in constant energetic motion within all things. It is the catalyst which creates motion in everything within the universe. Modern laws of physics support this ancient knowledge by saying that matter is just another form of energy, constantly changing in particles or wave forms.

*Qi is the mist that rises from earth to form clouds*

**Qi manifests:**
Physically as matter in the body

Energetically as resonant vibrations

Spiritually as divine light through infinite space

Morally as virtuous, conscious behaviors

Daoist practitioners cultivate an awareness of chi and it's pathways in many ways. Qigong and meditation are the most common ways. However, any conscious behavior that is aligned with Nature will assist one to develop an awareness of chi and learn to harness it's healing and creative powers.

The first step toward health and immortality is to develop your lower Tan Tien, the home of Jing. Picture 3 empty balloons stacked on top of each other. Your lower sea of chi, or elixir field is at the bottom of the three balloons, below your diaphragm. It is a big empty field, a sphere. With focused breathing and meditation practice you can accumulate and store chi in this lower elixir field, and that will concentrate to become a ball of chi in the lower tan tien. When a ball of chi forms in the lower elixir field to become a tan tien then you can circulate this ball of condensed chi along the meridians of the microcosmic orbit. This will harmonize and balance the jing chi and shen.

Exercises like tai chi, tan tien qigong, and specific breathing techniques will strengthen the lower field. Reverse breathing, or embryonic breathing, which requires you to pull up the pelvic floor on the inhale, and drop the diaphragm on the inhale to concentrate the chi in the lower field creates internal chi pressure in the lower elixir field. This is the opposite of Natural breathing.

To achieve a balance and create your foundation for long life you must, repair and Conserve a quantity of jing, Nourish quality of jing chi and shen, Store jing, circulate chi, Transform essence and chi to Shen.

Typically one strives to repair, nourish and stabilize jing and chi in the spring. In fall, harvest, repair and nourish to strengthen the lungs. Store and circulate jing and chi in winter.

**What is Leading? Jing Chi or Shen**
What do I mean by leading? What is leading your personal evolution? Body, Mind or Spirit? Jing, Chi or Shen?

We age thru the Jing. If the organs are not anchored in the body, then life becomes hard, and there are diseases and imbalances. Therefore, to achieve health and longevity one must take care of the body as it is the intermediary between heaven and earth.

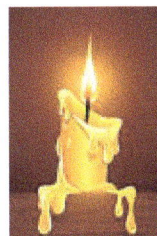

# Tao te Ching

Tao, a path or the Way. The mystery of all mysteries.
Te, virtue and virtuous application of subtle knowledge
Ching, a sacred text or spiritual guidance

*Tao is the Mystery of all Mysteries; un-namable yet all pervasive.*

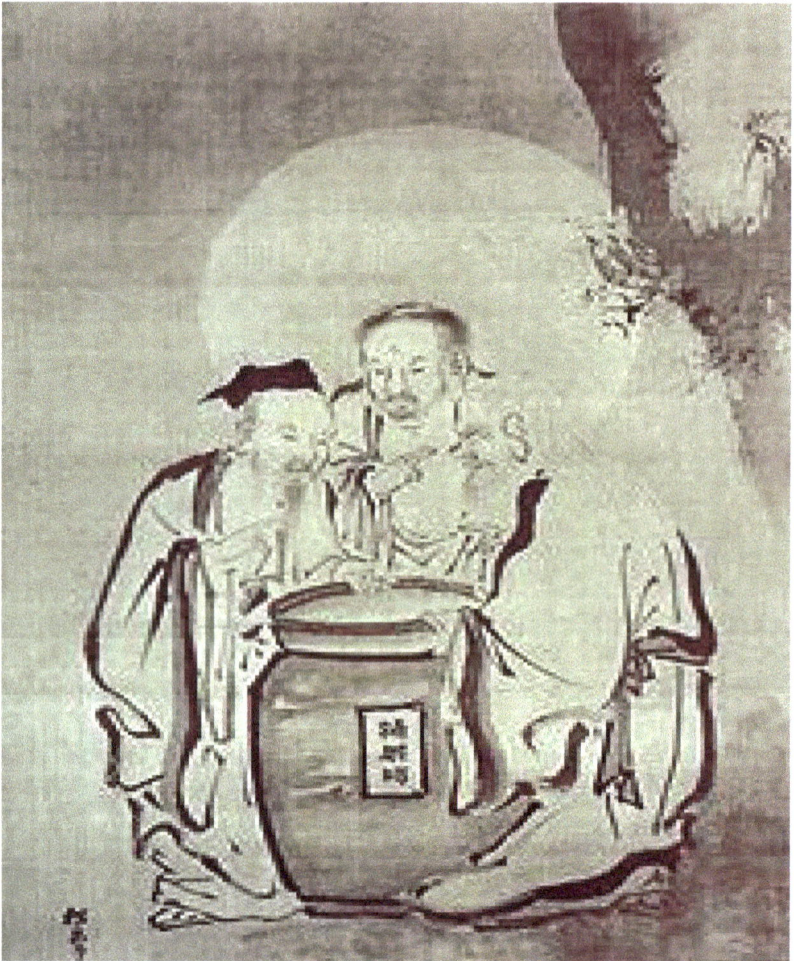

The Vinegar Tasters. Lao Tzu, Confucius and Buddha

Lao Tzu wrote the Tao te ching over twenty five centuries ago as a handbook for leaders and Taoist thinkers. In ancient China rulers were seen as the intermediaries between Heaven and Earth, and therefore, to lead wisely meant to live wisely, to seek personal balance, to honor and be observant of nature, and to keep sacred rituals alive.

Lao Tzu, (Li Erh), who lived between 570 -490 BC, wrote the Tao te ching for potential rulers who would be concerned with the correct Taoist way to rule. He was the keeper of the ancient Imperial archives during the Chou dynasty and was well versed in the wisdom and knowledge of China's sages. His official position in the government was historiographer, and he was also in charge of observing celestial phenomena and consulting the I Ching for the imperial court. It is told that he saw a time of great confusion and spiritual disintegration about to come, and because of this he decided to leave society in search of harmony with nature. He rode west on a water buffalo. As he arrived at the Western Han Gu pass the border official asked him to write down the essence of his wisdom. The border guard had observed a purple cloud following this mysterious traveler and knew that an important being was about to arrive. Lao Tzu agreed to write what became a famous treatise on Daoist philosophy in 5000 words.

Composed of 81 chapters, which read like poems, we are led into concepts which guide us in the ways of deep personal, political and spiritual contemplation. Like Sun Bu'er, the simple poetic rendering of deep thought opens our imagination and an ability to visualize complex advice.

One of the most sacred texts in Taoist philosophy, the Tao Te Ching has been translated more frequently than any other text except the Bible. Silk manuscripts and bamboo slips from the ma-wang-tui tombs were uncovered in 1973 in south central china (near Changsha) dating from 168 BC. From these archeological finds new translations, missing lines, vocabulary and grammar from the Tao te Ching were introduced to the public.

The "Way" is like a great womb, empty yet full of all things yet to become manifest; a symbol of all and nothing, having no real name. The Way is present in all things as chi, that infinite invisible unified pattern which manifests in physical reality. The Way of things is generally what Daoists mean by "virtue"; te. Te could mean virtue such as morality and right behaviors in society resembling the teachings of Confucius.

The Tao te Ching shows up in the section of Immortality practices to provide you with deep contemplation on the Way of things, including your place within all things. The point of view that we hold about life may guide our experience of life and our choices in response to what life presents to us. Some people study this writing their entire lives. In fact, Confucius visited Lao Tzu to seek his advice. After meeting with him, Confucius told his students that he had met with a Dragon, that mysterious ethereal being that flies to the clouds. He was saying the Lao Tze is truly the Old Master, beyond the average human in understanding of how the universe moves. The Tao te Ching is a contemplative and poetic book which can guide us to discovering an inner peace with nature, harmony within ourselves, and outer peace as it is applied to political trends and world patterns. I recommend that you look for one or two translations that you enjoy; there are many.

The Tao te Ching is also a guidebook of metaphysical secrets, meditation instruction, guidance on leading people toward productive society, and ways to harmonize with nature. It is simple, yet profound, classic Taoist thinking. The women who study at the Kundao school in China are required to take 2 semesters of the Tao te Ching. I have included a few of my favorite chapters out of the 81. But don't stop here, there are many translations to discover, including Benjamin Hoff's "Tao of Pooh." Winnie the Pooh symbolizes the ultimate in innocent perception in the present moment, and being in a state of Wu Wei; emptiness or effortlessness where everything is possible and everything is accomplished. (read chapter 63)

*Chapter 1*
Tao is beyond words
and beyond understanding.
Words may be used to speak of it,
But they cannot contain it.

Tao existed before words and names,
Before heaven and earth,
Before the ten thousand things.
It is the unlimited father and mother
Of all limited things.

Therefore, to see beyond boundaries
To the subtle heart of things,
Dispense with names,
with concepts,

with expectations and ambitions and differences.

Tao and its many manifestations
Arise from the same source;
Subtle wonder within mysterious darkness.

# Taoist Dream Practice

# Cultivate your Spirit in Solitude

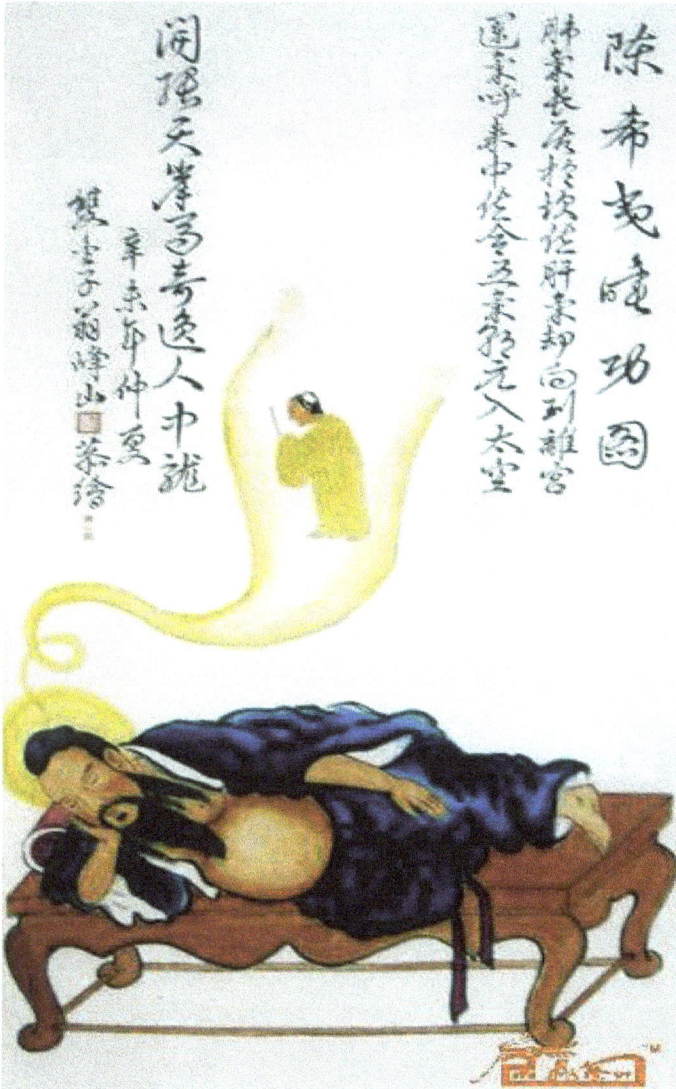

*Chen Tuan, The Dreaming Priest*      -Artist unknown

**History and Chen Tuan**

In the West we measure history in hundreds of years. The history of China is measured in the thousands of years and, therefore, the roots of Taoist Dream Practice fade into a mist of antiquity and mystery. Dynasties lasted for hundreds of years and endorsed practices that shaped the people and beliefs of the time. The Shang Dynasty which spanned the years 1600-1046 BC was the second official dynasty of China.

The stability of the country during the Shang Dynasty led to numerous cultural advances such as bronze casting, the calendar, religious rituals, Taoism, writing, and the I Ching. Recorded history tells us that the early Shang king worked for the people of his country instead of for his own pleasure and provided a role model for his successors. As was customary for the time, the imperial courts employed Sages, Shaman and Oracle readers to advise the king on personal decisions and in matters of ruling the country.

During this period of time Taoism was seen as a personal spiritual practice, rather than a religion, and there were many men and women living simply and quietly in the Sacred Mountains of China secretly refining their spiritual chi. Retreating from society was a requirement for the fine subtle energy practices that these hermits kept alive.

Chen Tuan was born in Shih Chuang (Sichuan) Province in the early Song dynasty (960-1279 AD) and lived for 118 years, from 871-989 AD. His parents died when he was a teenager and he left everything to the villagers and wandered the country and studied. His favorite books to study were the Book of Changes; the I Ching, the Tao te Ching, and the teachings of Chuang Tzu. These 3 books were referred to as the Three Scriptures of Mysticism.

His Inner Alchemical Soul travels which resembled sleeping meditations were gleaned from the visitations of 5 old men who appeared to him one night as he was reciting the I Ching. They had thick eyebrows and white hair, looked ancient and came regularly to listen to him. He decided to ask them who they were. "We are the dragons from the Sun-Moon-Lake of this mountain. Mount Hua is where you should go to live as a hermit." The 5 dragons carried him to Hua Shan Mountain and told him to stay inside, which he did for 100 days, practicing and reflecting.

The old men appeared to him as Dragons, and we know from many legends that Dragons are very good at sleeping.

His later years were spent at the Cloud Terrace Monastery at Hua Shan Mountain. I have visited this place. Hua Shan is a beautiful mountain and there are, to this day, hermits living on the mountain.

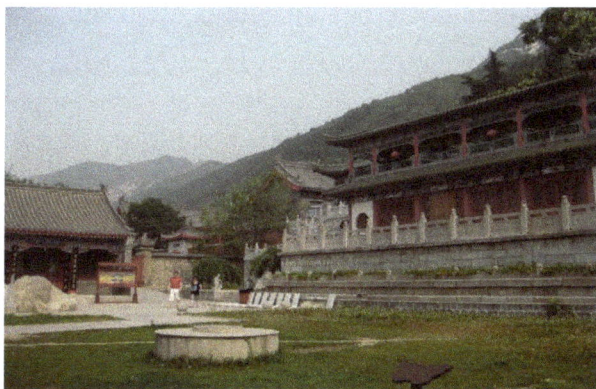

Cloud Terrace Monastery at Hua Shan Mountain, 2011

Chen Tuan became a wise man of great reputation, a Zhan Meng, who practiced dream divination and provided spiritual advice which directed political decisions during the Song dynasty. In 984 on one of his visits to the emperor he was awarded the official honorary title "Master of the Invisible and the Inaudible", Master of the Subtle Realms indeed! He regularly slept for months at a time. If one wanted an audience with Chen Tuan, the wait could be many days or months, as he slept.

One of his many gifts to the Chinese culture of his time was to influence Confucian thinkers away from the pursuit of governmental position, fame and glory and encourage them in the pursuit of the spiritual significance of life. Chen Tuan had no social ambition and although he was tempted by emperors he refused their offers in favor of his spiritual cultivation.

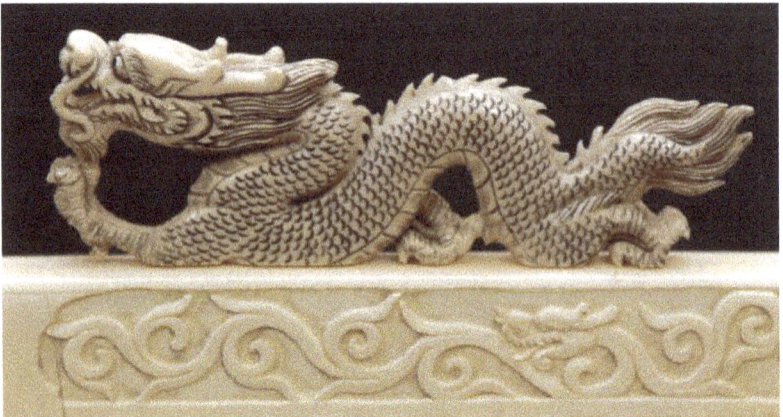

*He passed down 3 things:*
His achievement of the I Ching
His spiritual cultivation (Dream Practice)
His Tao Yin 24 postures

## What is Taoist Dream Practice?

Taoist Dream Practice is a Yin practice, (a creation practice). One cannot control the outcome. Dream Practice is accomplished by setting intentions, connecting with desire and surrendering. We prepare the mind, body and emotions, set our intention and let the seed take root. Preparation includes all of the finest basic Taoist practices such as Qigong, Inner smile meditation and the six healing sounds, moderation in eating and Tao Yin.

Chen Tuan's sleep was not the sleep and dreaming of ordinary people. His qigong practice is that of the 5 Hibernating Dragons. In the years that Chen Tuan studied the I Ching, he was most interested in the Pre Heaven arrangement of trigrams, that which represents the un-manifest and unseen. Pre Heaven is pure energy, the beginning of all things. His study made use of symbols and diagrams, such as the Tai Chi symbol seen below from Hua Shan Mountain. Taoist adepts study of symbols, diagrams and numbers is a classic method in interpreting the wisdom of the I Ching and the unseen realms.

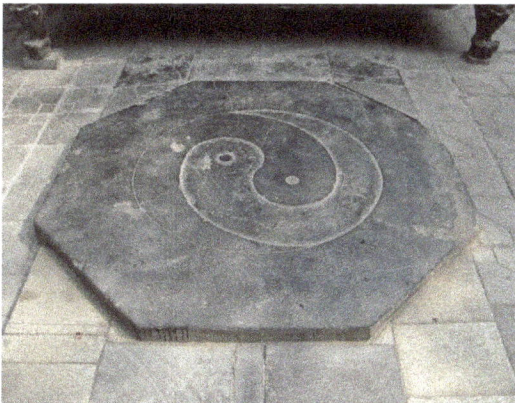

Stone Tai Chi from Hua Shan Mountain, 2011

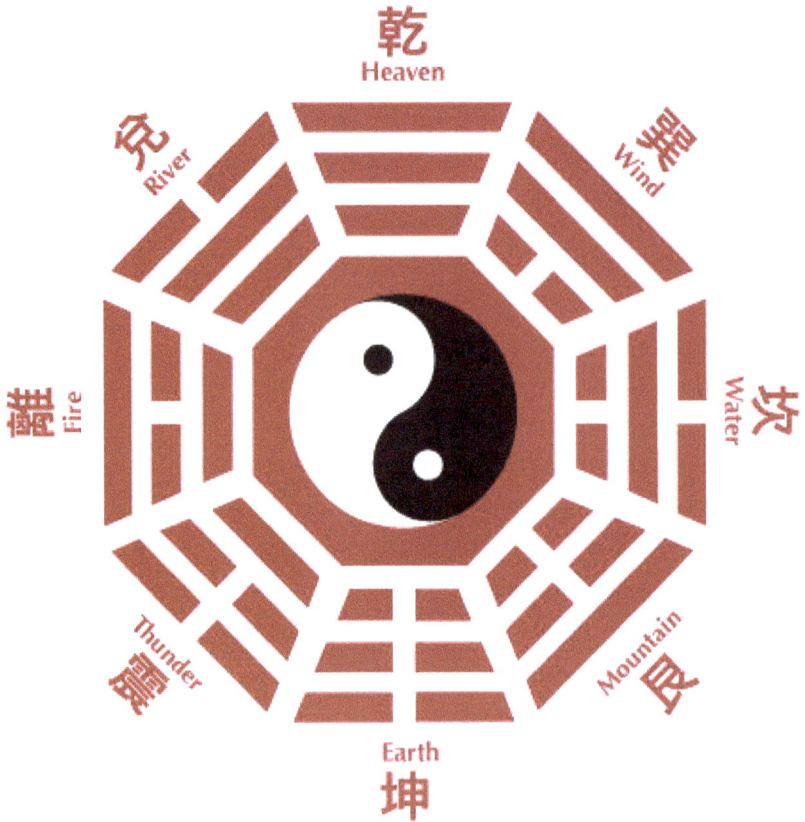

乾
Heaven

兑
River

巽
Wind

離
Fire

坎
Water

震
Thunder

艮
Mountain

Earth
坤

Pre Heaven arrangement of the Bagua

**(River also translates to Lake) Lines in a Trigram are read from the inside out.**

The most basic symbol used by Chen Tuan would be the empty circle to represent the un-manifest void. This is where everything, including our energy originates and where it returns. Many Taoist practices emphasize becoming familiar with your energy body and encouraging a conscious return to Primordial Chi. From the void is born Tai Chi, the union of opposites that sits in the center of the Baqua. Yin and Yang define each other; they are opposite but mutually complementary.

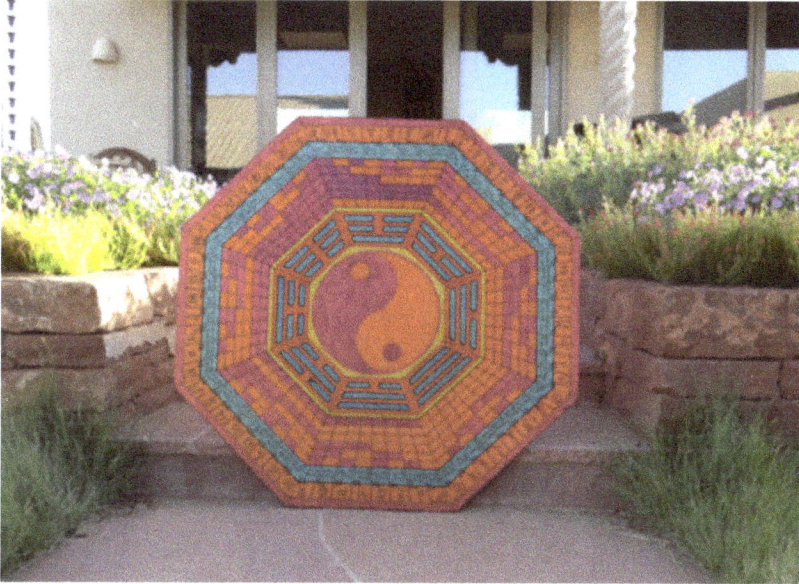

In this Pre Heaven Bagua you can see the dates of the Calendar around the outside in blue/green. The dark purple squares are yin lines. The orange squares are yang lines. You will find that the dates every year between December 18 and 22 in the Northern hemisphere include December 21, the winter solstice. This is a time of pure Yin chi, and the degree from North is Zero degrees. This is the direction one would face to pick up the energy of the time, exact North. This time period is represented by hexagram #2 of the I Ching; earth over earth; Kun. Pure Yin; the energy of responding, gentleness, waiting, bringing the seed into hibernation, devotion, humility and patience. The Solstices and Equinoxes are open gates for energy practices. Use these times as open portals, cosmic doorways, to potentiate your energy practices and to understand stillness within action. Chen Tuan understood action within his stillness in sleeping.

Our emotions and our 5 senses arise from within the body, and are also influenced from without the body. We digest life experiences like we digest food. Either we like the food or we don't, we feel content or we don't. Emotions are a daily activity of the organs and the senses. To facilitate a deep and peaceful life experience, and a restful and luminous sleep, we must digest emotions and bring our organs back into harmony each day.

We have been gifted with Taoist practices which were passed along orally over thousands of years, and finally reproduced in writing during the Han Dynasty. (206bc – 220ad) The Inner Smile and the 6 Healing Sounds are examples of Taoist practices which elevate the frequency of Chi in the physical body and the energy body so that we can achieve health, balance, harmony and a peaceful life. This quality of cultivated high frequency chi is the energy we take into our sleep and meditation.

We must harmonize our Dragon minds with our Tiger emotions, so that the energy body can refine itself; it is this level of consciousness that becomes immortal. Our Chi has a quality and a quantity that can is influenced moment to moment by our thoughts, emotions, foods, air, breathing, movements, environment, and intentions. When the body is at ease, the mind can also be at ease. This allows us to turn our attention to spirit.

There are times when we must simply sleep to keep the body healthy, and at these times we can enter into sleep consciously, with full intentions. Intention and Incarnation reside within the Central Channel; a deep level of our energy body/ chi field that is at a deep dimension of our being, deeper than ego and emotion. It is pure intention that holds us between heaven and earth. When our Central Channel is strong, deeply rooted between earth and heaven, we move confidently in life and bring into fruition our intentions.

Chen Tuan advised his students to abide with Nature and refine themselves even in sleep. As an energetic practice you will understand that your spirit, and energy, never sleeps, it is always active. Therefore, you can refine your energy as your body rests by setting your intention. Chen Tuan used sleep as a cultivation practice to nurture the "medicine of immortals." He taught his students to focus beyond worldly life to deeply reach the vastness and profundity of universal life.

*Taoist Dream Practice is a Yin practice. It is a way to carry out energy/chi cultivation practices without the limitation of the physical body.* It excels in the Yin time of year, especially on Winter Solstice. One cannot control the outcome of this practice, but you can prepare your mind, body and emotions with basic Taoist meditations and then set your intention. Clear and conscious Intention gives energy /chi a direction, or a dimension in which to manifest. Intention begins most everything we do in life.

As you allow your consciousness to merge with the slowing movement of the season and the darkness of winter you naturally drop into the stillness of meditation. Nature rests, becomes still, regenerates herself and waits. We take our cues from nature and find a still point during the Winter. The water element teaches us stillness, gentleness and the ability to be in flow without pushing our will beyond our limits. So, with Dream practice we connect intention with the energy body.

As we fall to sleep our senses turn inward. The first sense to become quiet is smell, then touch, sight, taste and finally, hearing. And our consciousness shifts from the physical to the subtle realms. Brain waves slow from Beta (13-30 Hertz) to Alpha (7-12 Hz), then to Theta (3-7) and Delta (5-2).

*Be mindful of this slow down transition phase, feel and become aware of it, because at the first frontier between Alpha/Theta you will give a Dream Command to your energy body, specifically instructing the Central Channel to hold your intention.*

**If you have prepared yourself for a short nap or a long night's sleep by eating simply and not too much, doing the Inner Smile and 6 healing sounds, Tao Yin, and feeling deeply into your Central Channel of intention, then you are ready to issue a Dream Command.**

When you first begin to practice you may simply fall asleep because the body needs to rest and to heal. Remember this is a Yin practice. Let go of the outcome. If you do not have an excess amount of high quality chi then any practice will fall flat. You must have extra chi/ energy available for these types of advanced practices. If your body and mind are very tired and need healing, that is the first priority. However, you may set a gentle intention as you drift off to sleep that your body heal as efficiently as possible.

Begin with simple intentions, like "I will wake up feeling happy" or "I will wake up with a solution for this question." Or "I will wake up feeling rested at 7am"

**The Goal of Taoist Dream Practice is to enter the dream state deliberately, fully conscious.**

Let spirit and energy embrace each other. Let dragon mind and the tiger emotions become harmonious. This is a time of deep quietude. Chen Tuan wrote this poem:

> *The achieved one has no dreams.*
> *His dream is not a dream,*
> *It is a voyage to the high spheres.*
> *The achieved one and even the secondary achieved ones do not sleep.*
> *When he rests, he nurtures his energy,*
> *So the fire in the stove never stops.*
> *The medicine keeps being refined.*

The stove that he refers to is in your lower tan tien. Your breath fans the fire under your cauldron to refine, gather and condense a high quality of chi. In order to cultivate a high quality of chi we must harmonize the emotions and quiet the mind.

You will recall in the practice of the Microcosmic orbit meditation and Fusion of the 5 Elements that the Cauldron is the receptacle in your lower tan tien that creates the Pearl of cultivated chi which you circulate in the meridians. It is necessary to fully understand and carry out basic Taoist practices like Microcosmic Orbit meditation before you attempt advanced alchemical practices.

## Basic Terms and Concepts to understand

**Chi** - Life force energy. Chi is infinite cosmic energy, and can be purified, cultivated, circulated, stored, or projected for healing. The physical body is the densest form of chi. Qigong practice is a good way to feel your own Chi field and to become familiar with the subtle energy body. As I mentioned earlier in this text, many things affect the quality and quantity of Chi.

**Central Channel** - Also called the Hara line, the Central Channel connects you and holds your life incarnation between heaven and earth. This is a deep Meridian of creative energy which holds your life's intentions. You may feel it as a vibration, or hear it as a deep sound. With right timing, you send your conscious awareness into this level of creation. Intention is the Alchemy of Inner Fire.

**Inner Smile Meditation** - The inner smile raises the frequency of the cells in your body. Joy is a non-dual experience, it exists in a higher dimension that the emotions that arise from the organs in the body. As you raise the frequency of every cell you bring more vibration into the central channel. The Inner Smile is a classic example of a Taoist meditation. Simple yet profound.

### 5 elements and the organs' emotions

Below are 2 graphs which illustrate the elements and paired organs, and the higher and lower frequency emotions that are associated with them. The 5 elements found in Traditional Chinese Medicine is part of the creation story and part of the evolution of our bodies.

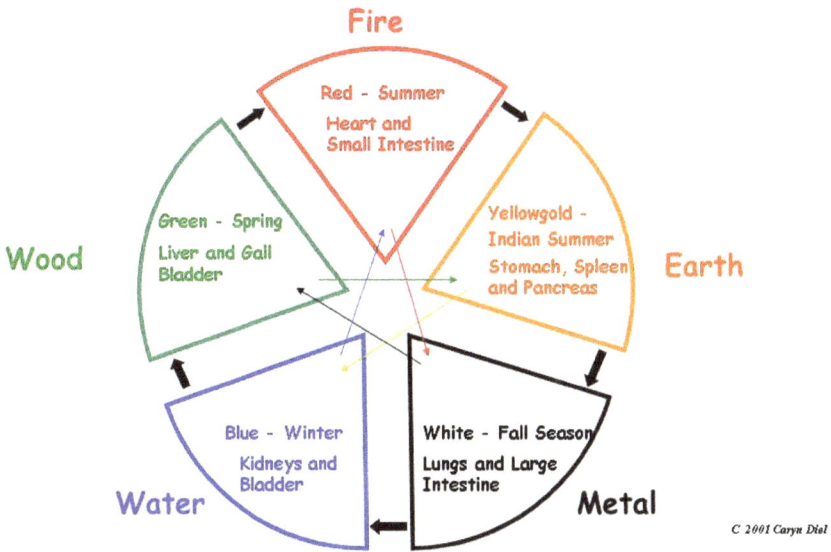

Fire
Red - Summer
Heart and
Small Intestine

Green - Spring
Liver and Gall
Bladder

Wood

Yellowgold -
Indian Summer
Stomach, Spleen
and Pancreas

Earth

Blue - Winter
Kidneys and
Bladder

White - Fall Season
Lungs and Large
Intestine

Water

Metal

C 2001 Caryn Diel

The arrows at the inside of the graph represent a Control Cycle. The thick arrows between seasons represent the Creation Cycle.

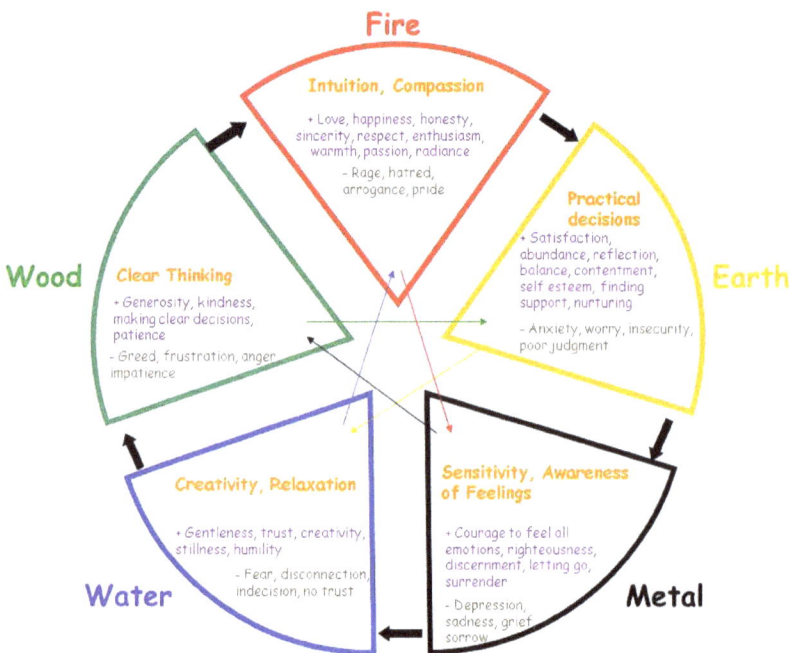

**Fire**

Intuition, Compassion

+ Love, happiness, honesty, sincerity, respect, enthusiasm, warmth, passion, radiance

- Rage, hatred, arrogance, pride

**Wood**

Clear Thinking

+ Generosity, kindness, making clear decisions, patience

- Greed, frustration, anger, impatience

**Earth**

Practical decisions

+ Satisfaction, abundance, reflection, balance, contentment, self esteem, finding support, nurturing

- Anxiety, worry, insecurity, poor judgment

Creativity, Relaxation

+ Gentleness, trust, creativity, stillness, humility

- Fear, disconnection, indecision, no trust

Sensitivity, Awareness of Feelings

+ Courage to feel all emotions, righteousness, discernment, letting go, surrender

- Depression, sadness, grief, sorrow

**Water**

**Metal**

C 2001 Caryn Dial

Here you see positive and negative emotions that are associated with the elements/organs. The words in Orange typify the behaviors or actions that would arise from the emotions. We sometimes refer to these as virtues. (the color of the Metal element is White, like the sun shining off of polished metal)

## Foundation Practices leading up to Dream Practice

Qigong and awareness of breath
Tao Yin
Inner Smile meditation
6 Healing Sounds
Awareness of Central Channel
Intention setting with Dream Command

*Qigong and awareness of breath*
Qigong has been practiced in China for thousands of years, and stands as one of the 4 branches of Traditional Chinese Medicine. There are many forms of Qigong, and all can be said to preserve health, cure disease, prolong life, develop strength, cultivate spiritual awareness and balance daily life, assisting us to find tranquility. Qigong practice is essential to longevity and will help you to bring more awareness into your Chi field through the intention of your breath and movement. The simplest form of Qigong that I know of is Shaking. Originally Qigong was called "dancing" and one may imagine the Shaman of old "dancing" around a fire until the Chi was flowing and the brain waves had shifted into Theta. Try shaking for 30-40 minutes and see what you experience. I have led groups in shaking Qigong at the summer Solstice around a fire pit under the stars and the results are very profound.

Remember to start your Qigong practice with long slow deep breathing and keep your movements slow so that you can feel and assess your chi field as you move. (Shaking Qigong may begin slow, but may speed up as you allow the chi to move on its own; it is spontaneous)

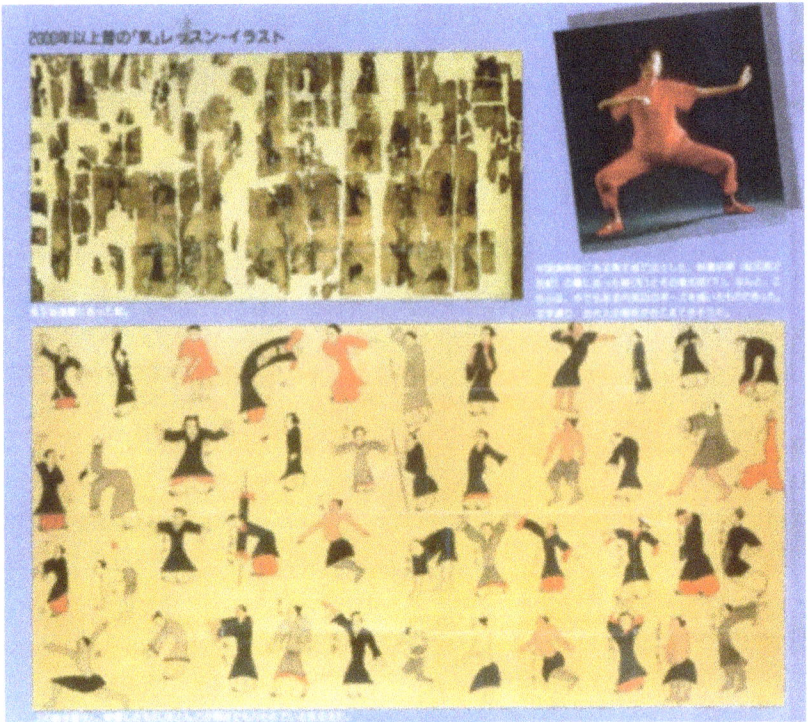

*Tao Yin; stretching open the meridians*

Tao Yin looks like Taoist Yoga consisting of stretches to open the flow of chi through the meridians. Hold the postures at a gentle stretch for three to five deep breaths which serves to extend the meridians and accelerate the energy flow. There are 12 ordinary meridians that correspond to the major organs in your body. They are located in the arms and legs and along the front and back of the body. Any stretch that you do will likely be affecting a meridian.

Begin with Conscious Breathing. Lying on your back, smile and breathe golden light into your entire body. Place your hands gently on your belly and feel the expansion of your breath.

Stretch out like a starfish with your hands above your head and stretch one arm, then one leg, the other arm, then the other leg so that you open the space around the kidneys. Feel the stretch coming from behind your navel.

*Kidney and Bladder Meridians*
Lying on your back. Bend knees, feet on the floor. Hug your knees into your chest, rounding the back to stretch bladder meridians along spine. hold and breathe Bring knees up toward your chest and reach thru to grab the ankles. Let the legs fall open to stretch the kidney meridian. Breathe 5 deep breaths.

Sit up with legs straight, and spine lifted up. Move your chin toward your toes to stretch the bladder meridian that runs down the back of the legs. Hands rest on top of the legs, do not round your spine, the entire stretch is at the back of the leg meridians.

*Liver and Gallbladder*
Sit with both legs extended straight to the front, opened as widely as is comfortable in a V. Do not raise the knees, but keep them attached to the floor. Keep the spine erect (not rounded) and reach forward until you feel a stretch in the liver meridian. If your hamstrings are tight you will feel this stretch simply by sitting up tall and not reaching forward at all.

Lying on your back again, bring the knees up to the chest, hug them in and then let them fall to one side, stretching the GB meridian.

*Lung and Large Intestine*
Sitting, clasp hands together behind the back and lean back, looking up. Then come forward bending to the floor with the arms and shoulders opening forward, hands are still clasped. Change thumb position and try it again. 5 deep breaths

Clasp hands, palms face sky, and reach over head stretching to both sides.

*Stomach and Pancreas*
Fold one leg in front of you and stretch one leg out behind you like a tail. Keep the spine moving forward. (pigeon pose). Change to the other leg. Take 5 deep breaths.

Sit on your folded legs, with the heels pressing into your bottom

*Heart and Small Intestine*
Sit with legs open wide, the knees bent and the soles of the feet together. Hold the hands around the toes, and bring the feet in toward the body as much as possible. Then, slowly bend forward trying to touch the forehead to the thumbs. Energy and blood are streaming toward the heart and small intestines.

Any other stretch of the arms that you enjoy will affect the heart meridian

*Hip Opener*
Cross your legs and cross arms with hands on the knees, bend forward toward the floor. Breathe. Change the leg and arms positions, to fold over again.
Gently shift awareness into the Inner Smile and 6 healing sounds meditation.

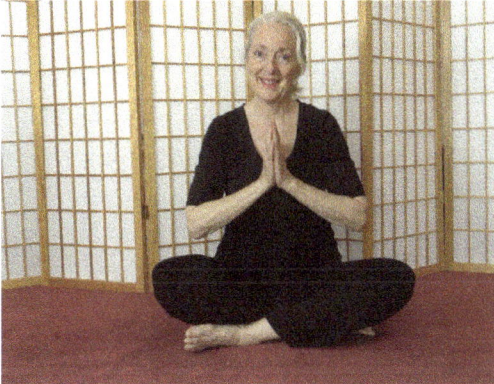

*6 healing sounds meditation; harmonizing the emotions*
Sounds and colors are used in the 6 healing sounds meditation. Sound and Color are ancient archetypes of healing. Sound breaks up stagnation and patterns of disease, in this case stuck emotions. Color tonifies the cells of the body. True colors signify vibrant health. See the above 5 elements graph to see the colors. (the Metal element color is White)

We begin the 6 healing sounds meditation with the Inner Smile practice which lifts the frequency in the cells to a higher vibration. Then visualize each organ filling with a pure color that is associated with it's element. The sounds will purge any low vibration emotion from the body. (the sounds are always sub vocal, like a whisper) For the Fire element the sound is

Haaaaa. Feel the sound emanating from the heart and small intestines, removing stagnation. The sound for the Earth element is Hoooooo, very guttural. Metal element sound is Ssssssssss. Water element sound is Chooooooooo, like a wave crashing. Feel the contraction in your core around the kidneys as you make this sound. Wood element sound is Shhhhhhhh. And the 6th healing sound is for the Endocrine glands; pituitary, pineal, thyroid, thymus, adrenal, pancreas, ovaries and testes. The color with will tonify them is a deep night sky violet/purple. The sound is Heeeeeeeee. The virtuous behavior that comes from balanced endocrine glands is effortless and harmonious communication.

Do this meditation daily before sleeping to clear your body/mind of low vibrations.

A typical practice session would be to begin with some Qigong movements, followed by Tao Yin stretching to encourage chi flow in the meridians. As the body is now relaxed and oxygenated, and filled with fresh chi you will want to sit and practice the inner smile and 6 healing sounds.

*Feeling your Central Channel and setting your intention with a Dream Command*
Stand with both feet firmly planted on the earth and see/feel a central beam of light moving through you between the earth and heaven. Taoists will point their heavenly energy toward the Pole Star. This engages 3 elements that are needed to create anything; this is the creative energy. Like a trigram; heaven, earth and humanity in the middle. When I say earth and heaven I am referring to dimensions. Human beings live within the dimensional energy of the physical earth that we

and all of nature live on and heaven, or the space that we see above and around us. When we meditate we refine our spiritual, non-physical energy, into the dimension of physical matter. This is the Alchemy of practice.

When you feel that you have made a connection to your Central Channel there will be a deepening of your awareness and a lack of ego and emotion. This dimension of your being is pure intention. Intention gives the creative energy a direction. Take a few steps, slowly, and feel your central channel moving with you. Is your central channel consistent along the length? Or is there more integrity above you or below you? The central channel is a deeper dimension than the emotional body. Your incarnation (en-flesh-ment) began at this dimension, and the emotions were experienced later as you were exposed to many life situations.

Feel into the vibration of your Central Channel as you are falling to sleep. At the border between Alpha and Theta you will send a non-verbal intention into your energy body. Keep it simple at the beginning. And let go of any outcomes. Remember, this is a Yin practice which requires patience and trust.

After a long sleep, Chen Tuan would stretch upon awakening. I recommend stretching and some self, chi massage. You have just done a long meditation.

**Here are the recommendations for your Dream Practice preparation.**

*Week 1*

Inner smile and 6 healing sounds before bed. Keep a sleep journal

Week 2
Qigong, Inner smile and 6 healing sounds before bed. Keep a sleep journal

*Week 3*
Qigong and Tao Yin, Inner smile and 6 healing sounds. Keep a sleep journal

*Week 4*
Qigong and Tao Yin, Inner smile and 6 healing sounds. Feeling your central channel and setting your intentions as you fall to sleep. Keep a sleep journal

Please contact me if you have questions or want to share something that you are experiencing. In the 3 weeks leading up to working with your central channel and the dream command, you can investigate what your deeper intentions may be for this time in your life. Also, if you would like a CD recording of the Inner Smile and 6 Healing Sounds meditation, I have one available on my website.

**Going consciously into the Dark time of year**
Winter season brings many gatherings and celebrations of all kinds. Our attention is scattered in many directions which may create stress. Please try to simplify your schedule during the winter months, especially leading up to the Winter Solstice. Taoist Dream Practice is an excellent way to harmonize your mind and body during this time. Try to limit the amount of time that you use electronics and artificial lights. Spend a day

without any of them. Experience the true light and dark of the day and night. In the Pacific Northwest the sun sets at 4:30pm, so there is a lot of dark time to be still and quiet.

If you are able to sync with Nature and slow down, your body will refresh itself and when the Light returns in Spring, you will feel a natural rising up of your energy. You will be replenished deeply from the winter rest and stillness.

*Simplicity and Stillness are the goals of the Tao*

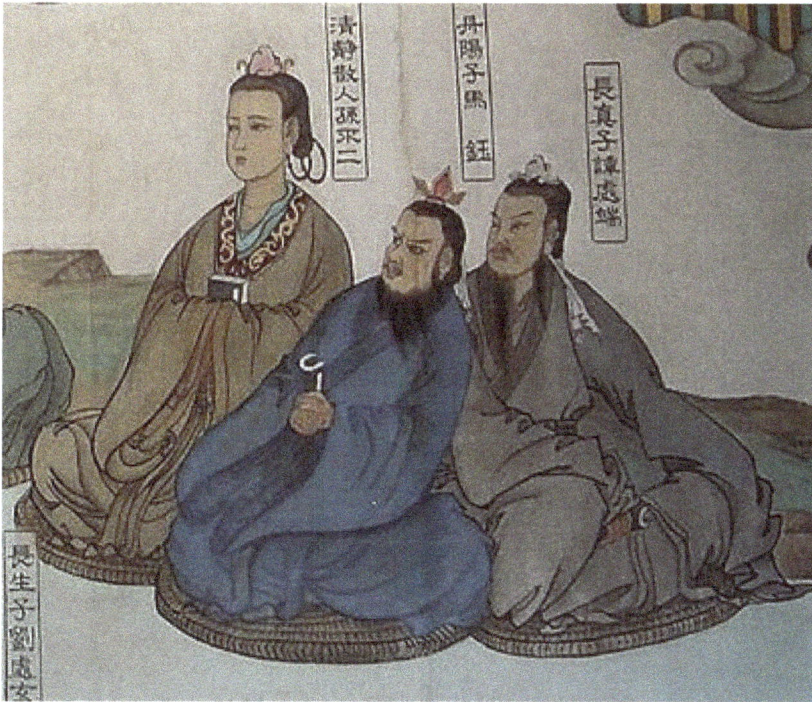

# Sun Bu'er

Sun bu'er is of the seven perfected (the only woman), of the Northern Complete Reality Daoist School in China. She lived between 1119-1182 C.E. in the Shandong Province of Northern China. The Complete Perfection, also called Complete Reality, lineage remains the largest Daoist organization in China today. The Northern Daoist School of Complete Perfection was founded by Wang Chongyang during the Sung dynasty around 1150 CE. He had seven disciples who became known as the Seven Perfected. One of his disciples, Ch'iu Ch'ang-ch'un created the Dragon Gate (Lung Men) sect of this lineage and took up residence at the White Cloud Monastery in Bejing. After her teacher's death Sun Bu'er moved to Qingjing and created her lineage, named Clarity and Stillness. She was given the title of Clear and Calm Free Human. She also studied with an advanced immortal sister who was a direct disciple of one of the teachers of Wang Chongyang. Sun Buer made use of the term *Kundao* designating the way of women in a Daoist context. The word Kun comes from the I Ching and represents Earth trigram, and the feminine principle.

Her cultivation instructions were written as poetry to describe her progress, including obstacles, towards immortality. Many Daoists write poetry as a way to teach. From a Daoist perspective poetry is the clearest vehicle for transmission of the multilayered knowledge of the Dao. Sun Buer was a Daoist Master and teacher. Much of her work reflects this style of teaching the Dao within poetry.

Her 14 poems lead us into the world of Daoist practices for women and give us some clues about the subtleties of internal cultivation, advice which is still pertinent today. She also composed a number of other poems which discuss inner alchemy for women and left three texts, one of them, *True Scripture of inner experiences of Jade like Purity*, which is said to have been handed down by the Celestial Mother of Violet Light.

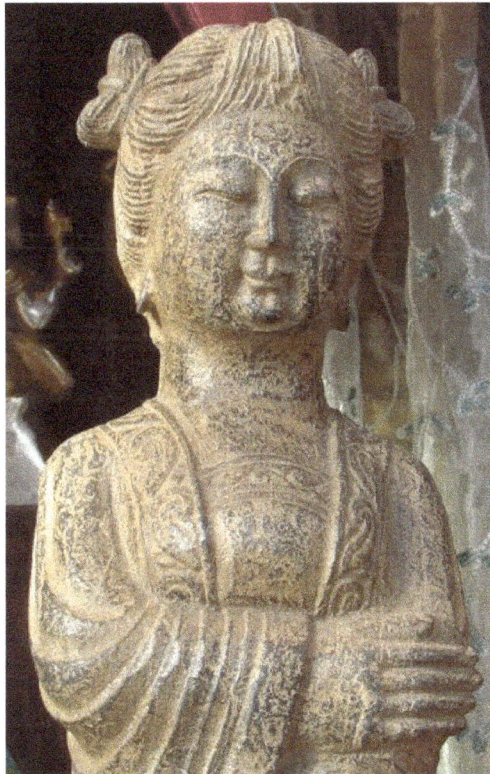

"Brambles should be cut away,
Removing even the sprouts.
Within essence there naturally blooms
A beautiful lotus blossom.
One day there will suddenly appear
An image of light;
When you know that,
You yourself are it"

Sun Bu'er. Translation by Thomas Cleary. *Immortal Sisters.*

Many times over Sun Bu'er advises us to simplify and unclutter our lives. Even in her time over one thousand years ago there were distractions. Imagine how she would see our busy lives today, with 5G and 24 hour drive through espresso stands. She had been married and raised three children. Her husband, Ma

Danyang, was also a student of the Wang Chongyang. Sun Bu'er began her Daoist training in earnest at age 51. She understood well the external demands of a householder's life, and in poem one, *Recalling the Mind*, she likens meditation to polishing jade to smoothness. "Sweep the space of the mind and clean up the ocean of thoughts." This is the first challenge faced by most meditators; to quiet the mind.

In poem two of the fourteen, *Cultivating Qi,* she lets us know that Daoist practice is a path of forward movement; once you begin to cultivate the Dao you will not want to come back. Sun Bu'er's poems reflect Taoist spirituality which holds that the cyclical changes in the human body and cycles of the seasons of nature world are related.

**The Kundao in Modern China**
Kundao in China today is a respectful way to describe a female Daoist who has left her family to study and live at a temple or monastery. *Kundao* combines two terms: kun and dao. Kun comes from the I Ching, and refers to Earth. *Dao* is the "way" which has many meanings.

In Nanyue there is a Kundao college, which was established in 2005. This Kundao school in the Daoist temple of Nanyue, (the southern marchmount of the 5 sacred Taoist mountains), is a two year program. Part of the Chinese Daoist College (Zhongguo Daojiao Xueyan), the first class of 48 females graduated on June 25, 2007.

The mission of this first Kundao class is summed up in eight Chinese words: Honoring Dao, Respecting De, (virtue), Learning and Cultivation, Progressing Together.

I visited the Kundao in their new location, a large elementary school, which they are renovating. Upon graduating the students will return to their original temples to become the leaders who will manage a modern temple.

The great merits of the female deities in each generation provide examples and encouragement for female practitioners. The encouragement and guidance of both the ancestral and fellow practitioners adds spiritual motivation for the growth of young Kundao.

The spiritual merit and the growth process of today's Kundao (women students at the College in Nanyue) are the image of growth and the changing history of women in new China.

I attended a conference in China in 2011 which focused on Women in Daoism. Wu Chengzhen, the Abbess of Changchun guan and chairman of the Hubei Daoist Association, spoke about the legacy of Sun Buer. Wu Chengzhen is the first principal abbess (Fang Zhang) of a Taoist temple in history. On Nov 15, 2009 her intense piety earned her an appointment as principal abbess of Wuhan's Changchun Temple, making Wu, age 52, the first woman to hold such an eminent position in China's only native archaic religion. She also spoke about the influence of "superior heaven and inferior earth" as a concept which influences women in China and how they are respected in Daoism. She made reference to the I Ching and the Tao te Ching.

#28 Tao te Ching
"Know the male,

Yet keep to the female;
Receive the world in your arms.
If you receive the world,
The Tao will never leave you
And you will be like a little child."...

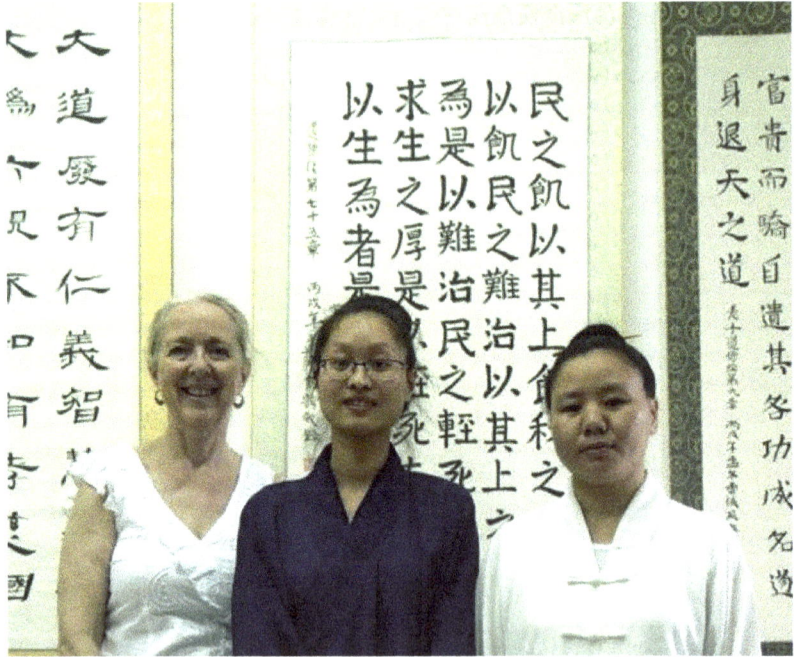

Author with female kundao students from the school in Nanyue, 2011

There have been women living peacefully and quietly in China's temples and mountain caves for centuries. Now, women have the opportunity to be formally educated, if they choose. They are learning to cultivate the whole person, and are currently playing a major role in the preservation and evolution of the Daoist temples in China.

**Poem #1 by Sun Bu'er**

*Gathering the Mind*

Before our body existed,

One energy was already there.

Like jade, more lustrous as it's polished,

Like gold, brighter as it's refined.

Sweep clear the ocean of birth and death,

Stay firm by the door of total mastery.

A particle at the point of open awareness,

The gentle firing is warm.

Page 7 "Immortal Sisters" by Thomas Cleary

She points out the fact that we existed as chi, energy, long before our body existed. As we seek tranquility through meditation we begin to polish our spirit like jade, and refine our essence like gold. Jade represents Yin and gentle concentration. Gold symbolizes Yang and intense concentration.

"Sweep clear the ocean of birth and death"; get rid of random thoughts. Forget past and future, Stay present in the moment.

**Poem 5**
*Cultivating the Elixir*

A very important difference between alchemical practices between men and women is this, women focus on the sternum, CV 17 point, while men focus on the lower tan tien. Bringing your attention to the location between the breasts in a critical instruction that has been left out, or lost, from most practices. Women's practices have been nearly lost over time, and so teachers have led women into practices that were designed for men.

**Poem Ten**
*Nourishment*
Cultivation is like a huge smelting operation
One can turn things into a mountain or lake.
The process builds upon a passion for transformation.
In the morning, eat the qi of the sun, like a turtle,
In the evening, absorb the essence of the moon, like a toad.
Gathering elixir astutely, the body feels light and lighter.
And when the original spirit visits
Ten thousand apertures emit a bright clear radiance.
Translation by Jill Gonet. Page 23 "Riding the Phoenix to Penglai".

There is so much advice embedded in this poem. Inner Cultivation is an alchemical operation which requires focus and right timing. In the morning look to the sunrise and gather in the essence of this time through the third eye, or Heavenly Eye. "Eat the qi of the sun like a turtle." Turtles have long been a symbol of immortality and can go long periods of time without eating food.

Begin to gather the sun's chi just before it breaks over the horizon and stop when it has fully risen. Do not look at the sun with your eyes open or you will injure them. To receive the sun's essence is a cultivation practice developed by ancient Daoist practitioners. The timing between 5-7 am and 5-7 pm is key to absorbing the chi of light from sun and moon. Your body is now digesting light energy. As you look into the center of the sun there is the presence of infinity which resonates with the infinity of your soul. The nourishment of sunrise practices stimulates your body to manufacture vitamins and minerals in response to the light coming into your eyes and into the pores of your body.

"Ten thousand apertures emit a bright clear radiance" Every pore in the body emits and gathers chi and light. Dawn, the time when everything awakens to life, is a symbol of yang and of creative, unmanifest potential. "In the morning, eat the qi of the sun, like a turtle, In the evening, absorb the essence of the moon, like a toad. Absorbing chi of the sun and the moon Sun Bu'er partakes of the inherent power of celestial bodies and feeds on the pure creative energy of the universe its most subtle form. " Gathering elixir astutely, the body feels light and lighter." In poem eleven she talks about fasting; a practice called Bigu.

"In general, to treat ailments practice right after sunrise and preferably when the weather is calm and mild. Sit up straight, face the sun, close your eyes, curl the hands into fists, and click the teeth nine times. Then visualize the scarlet brilliance and purple rays of the sun, pull them into the body as you inhale, and swallow them. Envision this healing energy entering the inner organ or area of the body that is afflicted by the ailment" Sima Chengzhen 647-735. Written during the Tang Dynasty.

Absorbing the Moon's chi is basically the same as absorbing the Sun's chi. As with all chi practices, once chi is absorbed, we refine, circulate and store the chi for health and long life.

*Titles of the 14 poems of Sun Bu'er*
1. Recalling or Gathering the Mind
2. Cultivating the qi or Nurturing Energy
3. Practicing
4. Taming or cutting off the dragon
5. Cultivating the elixir
6. Embryonic or womb breathing
7. Regulating the fire
8. Welcoming or Grafting the medicine
9. Refining the spirit
10. Nourishment or Ingesting the Medicine
11. Bigu; abstention from grain
12. Facing the wall
13. Companion or projecting the spirit
14. Lifting off; flying

Many of these poems apply to the practice of both men and women, and some of the lines are specific to women alone. One can see the progression of dedicated practice and internal cultivation by the title of the poems. Meditation practice begins with recalling the mind. Internal chi cultivation continues with more focus and dedication to breathing practices and fasting.

Sun Buer and her disciples established a Quanzhen community at the Cave of Immortal Maiden Feng. On the twenty-ninth day of the twelfth month of 1182, having predicted her own death, she washed herself, put on clean clothing, and came before her disciples. She recited a poem. Then sitting in lotus position, Sun Bu'er left her mortal body. Legend has it that at the moment of her death, her former husband Ma Yu (who was far away) saw her riding up to heaven on a five-colored cloud. He tore off his clothes and danced with joy, celebrating her accomplishment.

Ma Yu is not the only one to celebrate Sun Bu'er. There are shrines to her in some Daoist temples. During later dynasties, she appeared as a character in a number of famous plays and novels. Many Daoist texts refer to her as Primordial Goddess Sun and the Primordial Goddess of Clear Stillness, considering her to have transcended the human condition.

The Complete Perfection movement continued to grow after Sun Bu'er's death. Monasteries and temples were established throughout northern China, and within 100 years of Sun Bu'er's death, there were over 20,000 Daoist monastics, 6,000 of which are believed to have been women. The Complete Perfection lineage is the primary branch of monastic Daoism today.

*Sun Buer*

Be free from grief and
  anxiety.
A solitary cloud and wild
  crane beyond constraint.
Within a thatched hut,
Leisurely read the golden
  books.
Forests and streams outside
  the window,
At the edge of the rolling
  hills, water and bamboo.
Luminous moon and clear
  wind;
Become worthy to be their
  companion.
 – Louis Komjathy translation

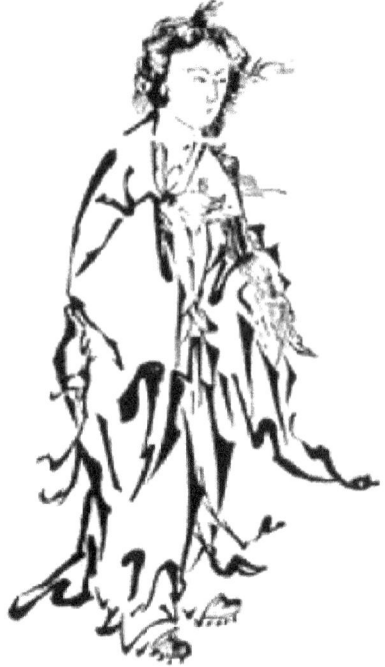

Throughout her life, Sun Buer was wife, mother, hermit, teacher, immortal, and goddess. She is an inspiration to all Daoists.

# Ho Hsien Ku

Ho Hsien Ku is one of the eight Immortals and the only female. The Eight Immortals were first recorded in the Yuan dynasty (1280–1368). They are said to bring happiness and luck. The Eight Immortals are a group of seven men and one woman who are said to have attained immortality. They guided and instructed each other in the ways of immortal practices.

Ho Hsien-Ku was believed to have lived in the 7th century during the time of the Empress Wu. As a child, Ho Hsien-Ku spent time on Yun-mu ling mountain. On this mountain there were stones called Yun-mu shih, "Mother of Pearl" or "mica." When she was around fourteen she had a dream. She was told that she must crush one of these stones and eat it so her body would gain great agility and be immune from death. Ho Hsien-Ku did what she was told and ate some powered mica. As a result of eating the mica she did indeed gain agility and immortality.

Every day she would go high up into the mountains and gather fruit to bring to her mother. As she was doing this, she found she was eating less and less. Eventually she gave up eating ordinary foods altogether because she realized she didn't need to eat in order to survive.

One day, the Empress Wu, hearing of Ho Hsien Ku, sent a message to have her brought to the palace to share her secrets of immortality. However, she disappeared from mortal view before she could be escorted to the empress. She is said to have been seen again in A.D. 750 floating upon a cloud of many colors at the temple of Ma Ku, the famous female Taoist magician.

Images of Ho Hsien Ku show her holding several items that are associated with Taoist immortality; magic fungus, a peach, sprigs of bamboo and pine, and flowers of the narcissus. Often she is shown holding a lotus blossom or wild fruit and herbs.

Fellow immortal Lu Dong Bin taught her internal alchemy, giving her a precious rare peach of immortality. Both he and Ho Hsien Ku are sometimes shown carrying a horse hair whisk which symbolizes their ability to fly through the air and walk on clouds.

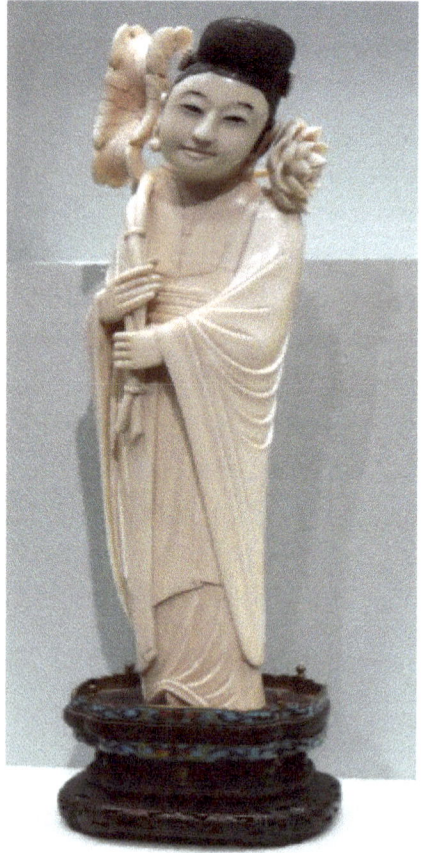

Ho Hsien Ku holding a lotus blossom. Symbol of open-hearted purity.

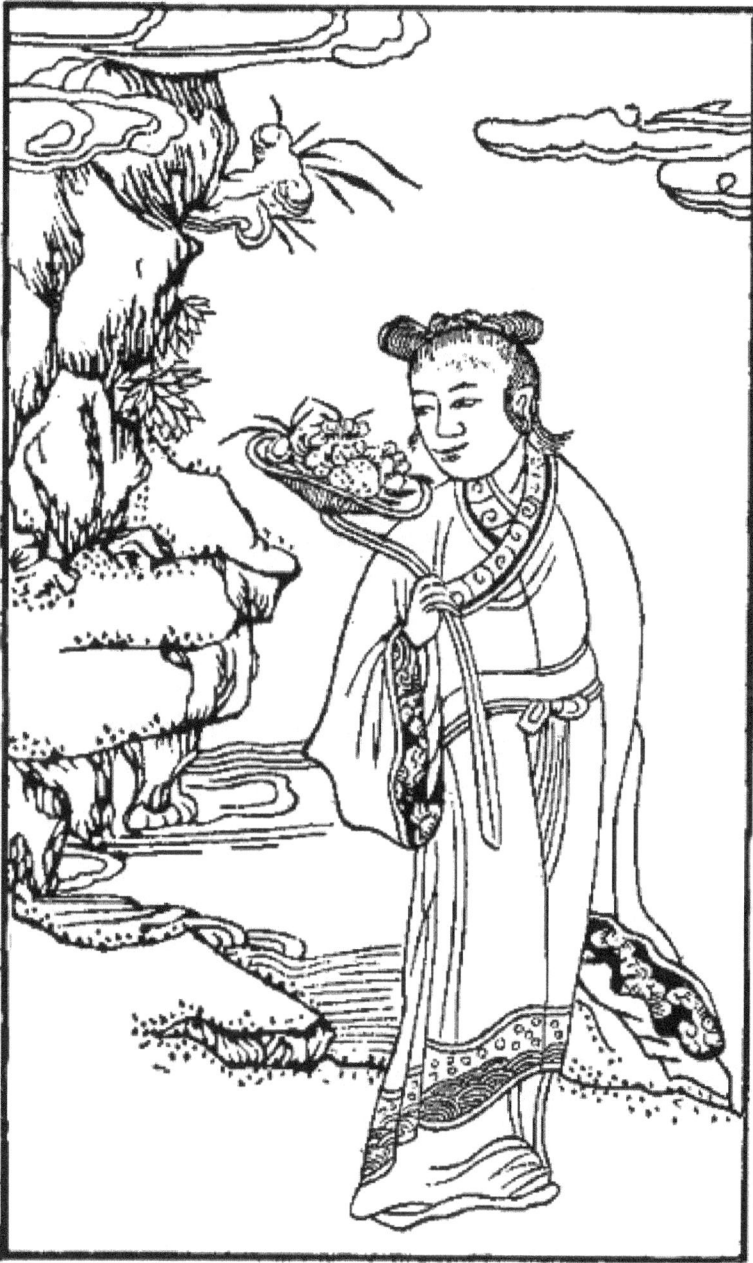

# Sun and Moon Meditations

The Sun and Moon have been revered by most civilizations on earth. Absorbing sunlight at sunrise and sunset will increase the frequency of your physical and energetic bodies. Sunlight has been proven to affect the production of hormones that direct our waking and sleeping cycles. The fire of the Sun produces all the minerals that our bodies need to stay healthy. Sungazing sets a harmonic resonance within the physical and spiritual levels of our being. Immortals, like Sun Bu'er and other masters, like Sun Simiao, developed their light body by sun gazing to such a refined frequency that they were able to live on sunlight, no longer needing to eat food.

It is recommended that you gaze at the sun just as it is coming up over the horizon, not starring into it which would damage your eyes, but gazing toward it and letting the sun shine onto your face. You can close your eyes. Your breathing should have the intention of absorbing cosmic solar chi on the inhale and gathering it into the deepest part of your bone marrow. Absorbing solar chi will help to regulate your blood flow and have positive effects on the heart. Stop Sungazing when the sun has fully risen. I have experienced an increased level of stable energy and steady deep sleep on the mornings and late afternoons when I have spent 10 minutes absorbing sunlight. The Daoist call this practice "heaven and humanity becoming one." It will repair the primordial chi in your postnatal body.

The Sun and Moon are a part of our personal Microcosm; our mirror of the universe. The sun represents yang, the moon represent yin. We are a harmonic balance of the two.

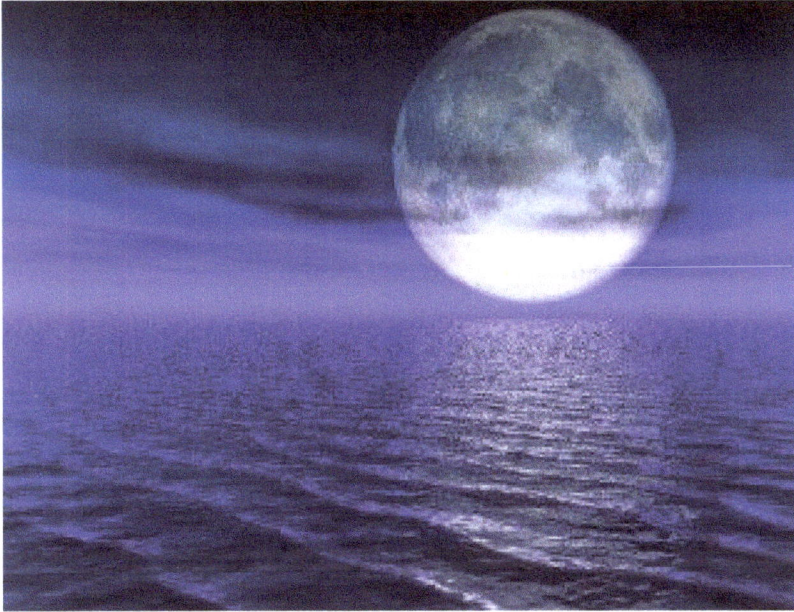

Absorbing the chi of the Moon is a process which involves absorbing and circulating lunar essence in the conception and governing vessels. It takes a little longer time to do this practice compared to the Sun practice. Known in ancient times as "immortal ascends to the moon." During the Full Moon stand comfortably in wuji posture and let your palms open toward the moon. Become still and breathe smoothly. Bring the moons light into your body universe. See your body inside the heavenly universe. This is where you begin. I find this practice to be very inspirational as it opens a deep connection to intuition and intention. The Moon's refection returns your shen inward, into self-awareness. The light of the moon is gentle and penetrating.

There are advanced practices for Sun and Moon meditations that need to be guided by a master teacher.

**Poem Ten by Sun Buer**
*Nourishment*
Cultivation is like a huge smelting operation
One can turn things into a mountain or lake.
The process builds upon a passion for transformation.
In the morning, eat the qi of the sun, like a turtle,
In the evening, absorb the essence of the moon, like a toad.
Gathering elixir astutely, the body feels light and lighter.
And when the original spirit visits
Ten thousand apertures emit a bright clear radiance.
Translation by Jill Gonet. Page 23 "Riding the Phoenix to Penglai".

# Endnotes

# Daoism in China Today

If one desires to become a Daoist in China today one first finds a local master, often living in a small temple. After some basic training and with family approval, he or she is officially adopted into a lineage, such as the Complete Reality lineage of Sun Bu'er and her school of 'Purity and Stillness'. Some adepts choose to live a celibate life at the monasteries and others live with their families in the community.

All schools and lineages follow a system of initiation and the giving of a spiritual name. Depending on the lineage chosen, each specializes in certain kinds of texts, rituals, and practices. Many modern day Daoists study with more than one master and hold the information of several lineages.

The White Cloud Temple in Beijing is a seminary for monks, as is a temple on Mount Qingchen. Nuns are able to receive Daoist training at a school and temple located at the foot of Nanyue, the sacred mountain of the south near Changsha.

"At either place, the course lasts two years, with classes of 50-100 students. The curriculum closely matches traditional Chinese education, being broadly oriented toward cultivating the whole person, not only conveying knowledge but also mental, spiritual, and physical discipline. Students are taught many subjects, including Chinese culture, foreign languages, and temple administration, as well as Daoist history, ritual, music, literature, thought, taiji quan, internal cultivation, and more.

After passing the relevant examinations, graduates undergo advanced ordination to receive further texts and extensive precepts, often a major central ceremony held at the White Cloud Temple. They then typically return to their home institutions and take on the responsibilities of managing them in a modern way. Some also remain in the capital and work for the Chinese Daoist Association or in government agencies. Usually aged between 21 and 35, the newly trained elite is set to become a vigorous force promoting the Party-approved development of Daoism in future decades." Livia Kohn, website blog.

"Kundao is a common name for the female Daoists in China today, but no one knows for sure how many Kundao there are. According to Wang Yier (the chief editor of Journal of Chinese Daoism) at the White Cloud Daoist temple in Beijing, half of the Daoists who are living in temples around China are Kundao. There are over ten thousand of them. The Kundao in many ways are more sincere and committed to their faith than their male counterparts. The significance of the Kundao is reflected in the existence of a Kundao school in the Daoist temple of Nanyue 南岳(South Mountain), Hunan. This two-year on-site program is a part of the Chinese Daoist College (Zhongguo Daojiao Xueyuan); its first class commenced on September 12, 2005 and finished on June 25, 2007. This Kundao class selected 48 female chujiaren from 32 temples in 16 provinces around China".

By Robin Wang
Loyola Marymount college
Private interview in July 2006

It takes great courage and will power for modern day Kundao to defy well-defined social roles and to pursue their faith, freedom and self-realization. In the past, women peacefully spent all their lives in the temples of the mountains. Qingcheng, Wudan, Nanyue and Huashan all have centuries old traditions of female Daoists living on the mountains. Today these female Daoists are given a unique opportunity to be formally educated and schooled. This opportunity is particularly precious for them, given that most of Kundao come from impoverished conditions with little chance for advanced education.

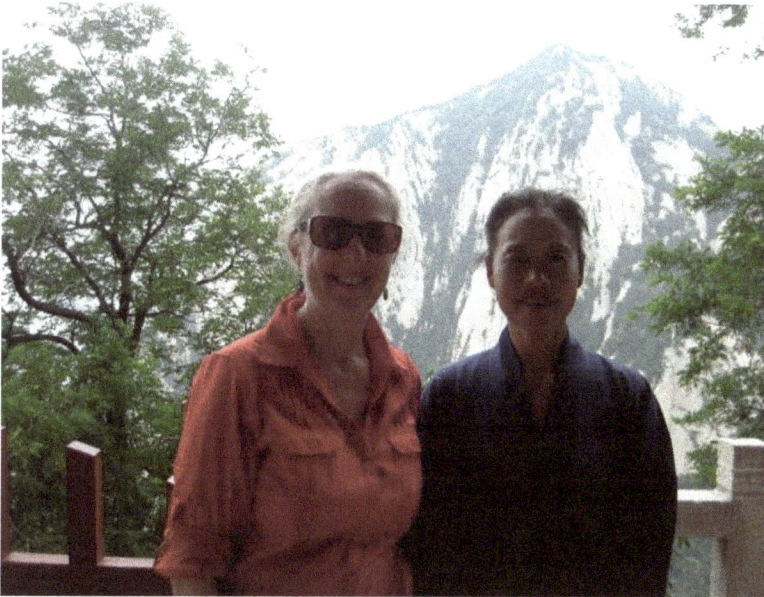

Me with female Daoist on Huashan mountain 2011

"For many centuries Daoist temples have been supported by local communities. For example, those who visited temple would bring sack of rice or other goods. Today China's free market economics and profit-driven tourism have brought up many difficulties for the survival of a temple in the mountains. Temples have to compete with local travel bureaus, which often charge large fees for entering the mountains, making worshippers less inclined to donate money to the temples themselves. How to manage and sustain a temple becomes a serious challenge for Daoists. In order to survive in this reality, these future Kundao masters must learn the skills of contemporary management and apply them in a Daoist context." Robin Wang, Loyola Marymount. Blog article.

# Practices for Girls and Young Women

Daoists see human development proceeding in five stages; young at age 7, sexually mature (leaking chi) at age14, damaged (from menstruation and childbirth) , declining at age 42, and weak or old at age 49. Prior to a girl reaching the age of 14 she is considered young which means that she does not need to do any special practices to cultivate her chi. Young girls naturally possess the foundation of chi that they need to stay healthy and vibrant. A female matures in cycles of 7 years. Boys mature in cycles of 8.

The Conception vessel and the thrusting vessels are responsible for regulating the changes in an individual's life cycle. For women those cycles occur every seven years. When these two vessels mature and fill with chi around age 14, the young girl begins menstruation. This is a good time to begin moon practices, as the menstrual cycle follows the cycle of the moon. Also a young woman can begin microcosmic orbit mediation to manage and balance her chi, and well breast massage to harmonize hormones and bring stability to jing chi and shen. Qigong and meditation practice is good at all ages.

When a young woman begins to have sexual intercourse her chi begins to leak and she must repair this with practices which strengthen blood and essence. Diet is especially important, as are meditation practices to harmonize the organs and emotions, such as the six healing sounds.

A young woman needs to learn to seal the 3 orifices of the pelvic floor to prevent leakage of chi. Start with breathing, and closing the earthly gate. Spend time walking in nature. Begin to understand Yin and Yang energy. Girls and young women should not try to emulate the yang masculine practices as this will harm their chi in the long run.

At age 42 a woman's chi is declining. At age 49 she is considered old. Older women in China are considered a treasure and birthdays are only celebrated once a person turns 49.

As we age we must practice longer periods each day to cultivate, store, strengthen and restore original chi. The body is the foundation for many internal alchemy practices, therefore one must nurture jing chi and shen.

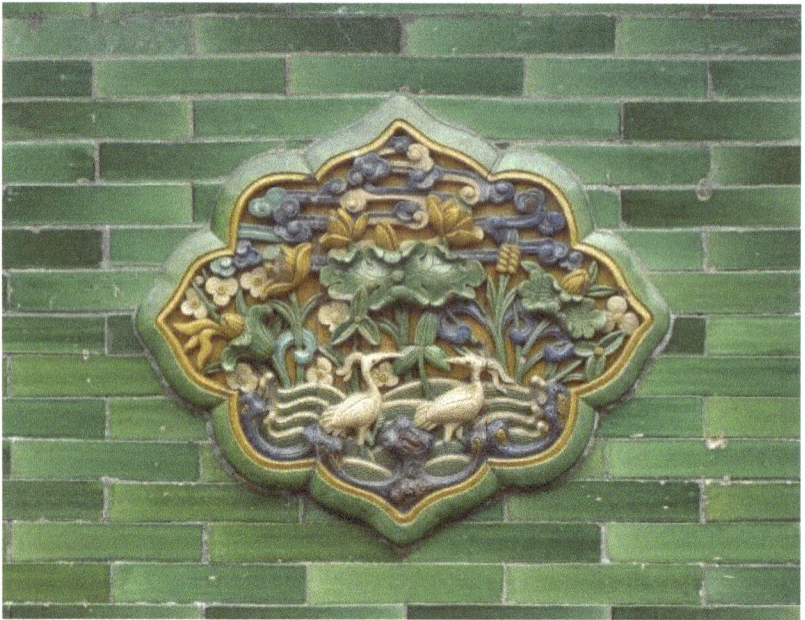

# ABOUT THE AUTHOR

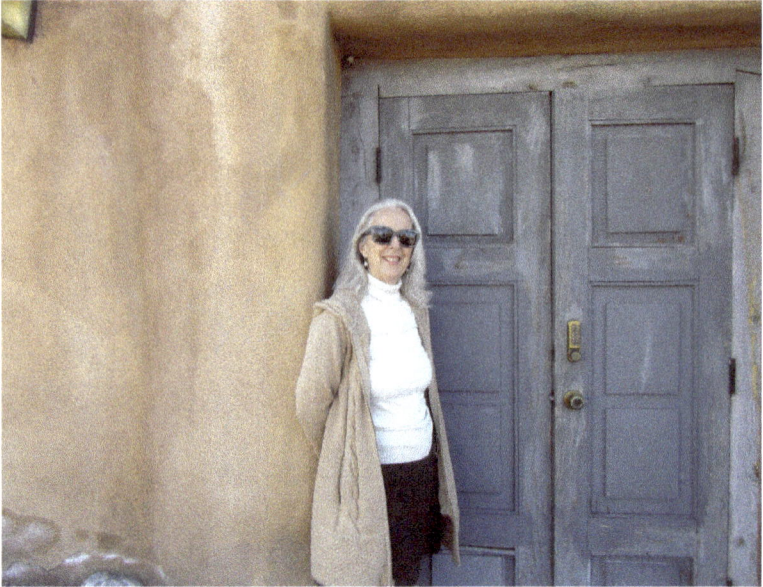

Caryn Boyd Diel is the founder and director of the White Cloud Institute. A graduate of the Barbara Brennan School of Healing and a Senior Healing Tao instructor, Caryn is able to move fluidly between the physical, emotional, mental and spiritual bodies to assist clients and students to find new direction and wellness. She brings a compassionate understanding to the journey of healing and self-discovery. Caryn enjoys teaching others about health and the evolution of consciousness. She combines cutting edge quantum physics with ancient Taoist teachings into her ever evolving curriculum. For more information on certification courses or continuing education visit the website; WhiteCloudInstitute.info.

Caryn has been teaching Healing Tao classes around the world for 20 years. She currently is a student of Nathan Brine in Vancouver, BC who has been trained in Taoist meditation and alchemy by Wang Liping.

www.ingramcontent.com/pod-product-compliance
Lightning Source LLC
Chambersburg PA
CBHW041219030426
42336CB00024B/3395